A Guide to
Personal Fitness Training

Revised Edition

by

Mary Yoke, MA

Editor

Laura A. Gladwin, MS

Published by
Aerobics and Fitness Association of America
15250 Ventura Blvd., Suite #200
Sherman Oaks, California 91403-3297
(818) 905-0040 FAX (818) 990-5468
www.afaa.com
afaa@pop3.com

  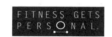 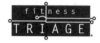

AFAA Fitness Practitioner, AFP Fitness Practitioner, Aerobics and Fitness
Association of America, AFAA and American Fitness are registered trademarks of
Aerobics and Fitness Association of America. Fitness Triage, Fitness Gets Personal,
FitMarkers and Fitness Management for Life are trademarks of Aerobics and
Fitness Association of America. Other names may be trademarks or registered
trademarks of other companies, and are used only for explanation and to the
owner's benefit, without intent to infringe.

ISBN 0-9614719-9-9

Printed in the United States of America
10 9 8 7 6 5 4 3 2

Contents

Acknowledgements

The editor wishes to acknowledge the guidance and talents of the following people in the creation of this book.

AFAA President: Linda D. Pfeffer, RN
AFAA Executive Vice President: Roscoe K. Fawcett, Jr.
AFAA Vice President, Educational Administration: Robin Foss
AFAA Board of Certification and Training:
Nancy Gillette, MA, Laura A. Gladwin, MS, Peg Jordan, RN, MA and Kathy Stevens

Editorial Production
Text Editor and Assistant Production Editor: Julie van Roden
Cover: Roscoe K. Fawcett, Jr. and Laura Carrington
Illustrations: Michael Aniel
Contributing Illustrators: Erin O'Driscoll and Laura Carrington

Reviewers

Wayne L. Westcott, Ph.D
Fitness research director at the South Shore YMCA, Quincy, MA.; strength training consultant for numerous national organizations, e.g., American Council on Exercise, the National Sports Performance Association and the National Youth Sports Safety Foundation; editorial advisor for *SHAPE, Prevention, Club Industry, American Fitness* and *Nautilus* magazine publications; author of several fitness books including, *Building Strength and Stamina* (newly released); recipient of IDEA's Lifetime Achievement Award and the Healthy American Fitness Leader Award, President's Council on Physical Fitness and Sports.

David Herbert, JD
Senior partner of Herbert Benson, Canton, OH; co-editor of *The Exercise Standards & Malpractice Reporter* and co-author of *Legal Aspects of Preventive, Rehabilitative and Recreational Exercise Programs*, 3rd edition.

Acknowledgements from the Author

I would not have written this book without a request from Linda D. Pfeffer, RN, President of AFAA, who originally asked me to write a workshop manual for AFAA. In addition, I owe a debt of thanks to Laura Gladwin, my tireless supporter and friend, who took on the daunting task of editing this book. I thank the entire AFAA board (members past and present) which has supported me and provided me with inspiration for several years. I would also like to thank Robert M. Otto, Ph.D., my earliest mentor in the fitness field, and an indefatigable source of knowledge and motivation for me. My thanks goes out to Larry DeLuca (AFAA Certification Specialist) who provided me with invaluable feedback as I was writing this book. I would also like to thank my parents, James and Margaret Yoke, who instilled in me a desire to learn, persevere and achieve.

About the Author

Mary Yoke received her Masters Degree in Exercise Physiology, and holds two degrees in music. She is an Adjunct Professor at Adelphi University on Long Island, NY, where she teaches a graduate course in "Techniques of Exercise Leadership and Functional Anatomy." She holds nine different professional certifications from AFAA, ACSM, and ACE, and has worked in the areas of cardiac rehabilitation, corporate fitness, the commercial health club setting, and as a physical therapy assistant. She is an AFAA Master Certification Specialist and Senior Trainer, and has presented on a wide variety of fitness and wellness topics internationally as well as in the United States. She is working on a new book entitled *Fitness Leadership*. Mary lives in New York with her two sons, Nathaniel and Zachary.

AFAA's Notice

This publication is intended to provide general educational information to assist fitness professionals, particularly personal fitness trainer candidates, in their efforts to obtain certification and in working with clients to reach definable goals.

This publication is written and published to provide what is believed to be accurate information. However, please note the following important cautions regarding the contents of this publication.

- To the best of the knowledge of the authors and publishers, the contents of this publication were accurate as of the date of publication. However, you are strongly encouraged to keep yourself informed of new developments in the field to make sure that the contents are still accurate when you consult this work.

- This publication is made available with the understanding that the authors and publishers are not engaged in rendering legal, medical, or other professional services by reason of their authorship or publication of this work. You are strongly encouraged to consult an appropriate legal, medical, or other expert if you are seeking such advice or assistance. This is an especially important precaution in the field of fitness and exercise, personal fitness training, and fitness practice.

- This publication is made available without warranties or guarantees of any kind. For example, the authors and publishers cannot and do not promise or guarantee that the contents of this publication are appropriate for every reader or user, or that use of this publication will result in certification or in obtaining employment as a trainer or other fitness professional; or that users, fitness professionals, or those who become certified will be able to obtain third-party insurance payments for any services that they may render to clients.

- The laws that define the practice of medicine or other health care fields reserved for those who are licensed to provide such services vary from state to state and according to specific circumstances. In some states and under some circumstances, the rendering of services may be actually or potentially in violation of law. For that reason, users are cautioned to obtain specific professional advice about the laws and regulations that may apply to them in a particular locality.

- The documents, forms, and other material contained in this publication are offered as illustrative examples only. No such documents, forms, or other materials should be used or adapted for use in violation of copyright or other applicable law. Since the use of these documents, forms, and materials may have legal implication, you are strongly cautioned to consult a qualified attorney before using or adapting them.

- This publication is not intended to establish or define any specific professional standards that apply to all fitness professionals and their clients in all circumstances or to limit the exercise of independent professional judgment by the user as to what is the best interest of any particular client. The standard of care which must be observed by a fitness trainer or other fitness professional may change from time to time or vary from place to place, and users are strongly cautioned to familiarize themselves with the standard of care that applies to them.

- All of these cautions apply to users of this publication regardless of their location. However, since this publication was prepared for use in the United States, special care should be taken by users outside the U.S. to make sure you are familiar with the laws and regulations that apply in your country and locality.

Part of the foregoing was adapted from a Declaration of Principles
of the American Bar Association
and a Committee of Publishers and Associations.

Foreword

Recognizing a vital need to set standards and guidelines applicable to personal fitness trainers as well as to provide qualified fitness professionals for Americans, the Aerobics & Fitness Association of America (AFAA) implemented its first national Personal Trainer/Fitness Counselor Certification program in October of 1990. The success of this program has been tremendous. Today, over 30,000 trained and certified personal fitness trainers have provided valuable knowledge, instruction, exercise programming and a professional standard of competency worldwide.

Personal training has come a long way—it is no longer just for celebrities. People of all ages, sizes, fitness levels and walks of life are enjoying the benefits of one-on-one fitness training. Today certified personal fitness trainers are working alongside health care professionals in health clubs, fitness facilities, hospital wellness centers and older adult communities providing the physical fitness component to lifestyle management. To stay abreast of their profession they are turning to a resource they can trust, *A Guide to Personal Fitness Training*.

A Guide to Personal Fitness Training was written to accompany AFAA's *Fitness: Theory & Practice* textbook. Together they provide the most up-to-date research and practical knowledge that have emerged over the past decade. Addressing wellness strategies, business ethics, exercise programming, fitness assessments, special populations, multi-training techniques and more, it provides the personal fitness trainer with a comprehensive textbook detailing the professional role for success in a very competitive and ever-changing world of personal fitness training.

Laura A. Gladwin, MS, AFP – Editor

Introduction
What is a Personal Fitness Trainer?

The field of personal fitness training is relatively new. As yet, there is no legal definition for a personal trainer. In some states, the use of the term "trainer" may, by statute or regulation, be limited to those who are licensed, certified, or registered by the state as such. In those situations, fitness professionals may have to qualify their use of the title or even select a new title under which to provide service. The advice of individual legal counsel in this regard may be appropriate. Practically speaking, however, most personal fitness trainers can be described by what they do—teach safe, effective, individualized exercises to clients in a one-on-one type setting. They assist clients in achieving the clients' personal fitness and wellness goals.

Personal trainers are responsible for screening clients and evaluating their ability to take part in fitness programs. These trainers have a duty to put safety first, to "do no harm." In order to follow this axiom, knowledge of industry guidelines for health screening and an understanding of injury prevention techniques are critical. To ensure the clients' welfare, personal fitness trainers need to recognize their own limitations and understand their scope of practice. Unless a trainer has specific training and/or licensure in subjects, such as clinical exercise testing and programming, massage therapy, physical therapy, chiropractic, and nutrition, he/she should be cautious of appearing to practice or give advice in these areas. Again, keep in mind that some states may prohibit the use of the term "trainer," at least without a qualifying statement.

Personal fitness trainers individualize exercise programs to fit client goals. In order to understand the client's goals and provide appropriate motivation and education over time, personal fitness trainers need to have strong communication skills and understand principles of long-term lifestyle change. In addition, a broad knowledge base is necessary to adequately answer (or provide referrals to other professionals who can answer) the many questions clients have about exercise, calorie expenditure, healthy eating, weight loss, injuries, and the like.

Personal fitness trainers recognize that one of their duties is to enhance clients' feelings of self-efficacy, the feeling of "I can do it; I am capable!" Teaching clients that they are responsible for their own health, that they can practice enhanced well-being, and that they can be independent are skills of quality trainers.

Personal fitness trainers must take seriously their responsibility to stay up-to-date on new research and medical findings. As the fitness field grows closer to medicine and science, trainers must continue to upgrade their education if they are to remain competent and perhaps to obtain required licensure, state-mandated certification, or registration when necessary. A great deal of misinformation and folklore is still promoted by some media and individuals as fact. A qualified personal fitness trainer has the knowledge and the ability to think objectively and separate fact from fiction.

In summary, a personal fitness trainer is a skilled teacher, motivator, communicator, and continual student of fitness and positive lifestyle change. Trainers serve a valuable purpose in helping people become healthier and happier, and in improving the quality of many lives.

1

Wellness Strategies

What is wellness and how can it be approached? Wellness, according to Dr. John Travis, MD, MPH, was envisioned by its originators as a multidimensional concept incorporating the mental, emotional and spiritual aspects of a human being. Wellness can be approached from at least two related perspectives. They are:

1. Prevention—the practice of behaviors that minimize the risk of lifestyle-related diseases and disabilities. One of the roles of a personal fitness trainer is to help clients identify risk factors and enhance well-being.

2. Holism—the integration of the mind, body and spirit for optimal functioning. Dr. Halbert Dunn identified five dimensions of the total person: emotional, social, intellectual, spiritual and physical. When these aspects are fully developed and integrated, optimal well-being results, which he called a "zest for living."

Many people associate wellness with fitness, nutrition, or stress reduction, but it is much more. It is the self-empowered practice of prevention and full development of all the dimensions of life. But remember, wellness is a process, a way of life; it is not a state that can be achieved once and for all.

The Wellness Continuum

| Disability | Symptoms | Awareness | Education | Growth |

Premature
Death

Neural Point
(No discernible illness
or wellness)

High Level
Wellness
(zest for life)

(Adapted from the work of John W. Travis, MD)

Good health depends to a great extent on the lifestyle choices we make, including what we eat, whether or not we are active, whether or not we smoke and how we manage stress. Many diseases and disabilities have been identified as preventable, or at least modifiable. One important role of the personal fitness trainer is to assist clients in identifying risk factors and practice prevention (see 1-8 below), helping clients to minimize illness and guiding them toward wellness. Emphasize to your clients that the same few risk factors influence several diseases and conditions.

Plan for Prevention

Condition/Injury	Diet	Exercise	Avoid Smoking	Moderate Alcohol	Control Obesity	Control Stress	Use Seatbelt
Heart Disease	✔	✔	✔		✔	✔	
Cancer	✔	✔	✔	✔	✔	✔	
Diabetes	✔	✔			✔		
Emphysema			✔				
Cirrhosis				✔			
Osteoporosis	✔	✔	✔	✔	✔		
Back Problems		✔	✔		✔		
Accidents/Injuries				✔			✔

(columns under heading: **Preventive Behavior**)

1. Prevention of coronary heart disease

Coronary heart disease (CHD), also referred to as coronary artery disease (CAD), is the leading cause of death in the United States and in most of the developed world. The three major cardiovascular disorders are heart attack, stroke and hypertension. CHD is almost always the result of atherosclerosis, or narrowing (hardening) of the coronary arteries. Atherosclerosis is a slow and progressive disease that gradually develops over decades. The rate of development depends on cholesterol and blood pressure levels, cigarette smoking, and other risk factors. Atherosclerosis of the coronary arteries can lead to myocardial ischemia, or lack of adequate blood flow to the heart muscle, which may then lead to a myocardial infarction (MI), or heart attack.

Stroke is often caused by atherosclerosis of the cerebral blood vessels. Stroke can also result from a cerebral embolism, in which a blood clot (embolus) lodges in a cerebral artery.

The tendency for hypertension may be inherited, but several lifestyle factors (e.g., excessive salt, fat and alcohol in the diet, cigarette smoking, obesity, physical inactivity and stress) strongly affect its development.

Currently, hypertension afflicts one in four Americans and, as a sub-group, one in three African Americans.[1]

Risk factors that predispose individuals to CHD have been identified and may vary slightly according to the source.

According to the American College of Sports Medicine (ACSM), CHD risk factors are:

- **family history**—heart attack, coronary bypass surgery, or sudden death before 55 years of age in father, brother, or son, or before 65 years of age in mother, sister, or daughter

- **cigarette smoking**—current smoker or those who quit within the previous 6 months

- **hypertension**—140/90 mmHg, confirmed on at least two separate occasions, or on antihypertensive medication

- **high cholesterol**—total cholesterol >200 mg/dl (5.2 mmol/L), or HDL of <35 mg/dl (0.9 mmol/L), or on lipid lowering medication

- **impaired fasting glucose**—fasting blood glucose levels 110 mg/dl (6.1 mmol/L) confirmed on at least two separate occasions

- **obesity**—Body Mass Index of 30 kg/m^2, or waist girth >100 cm

- **sedentary lifestyle**—persons not participating in a regular exercise program or meeting the minimal physical activity recommendations from the U.S. Surgeon General's report (active a minimum of 30 minutes per day)

ACSM also identifies one negative risk factor:

- high HDL—cholesterol >60 mg/dl (1.6 mmol/L)

2. Prevention of cancer

Over one million Americans are diagnosed with cancer each year.[2] According to current research, it is estimated that about two-thirds of cancers can be prevented. Preventable cancers include:

- Cancer of the lung—the leading cause of cancer death in both men and women. The primary cause is cigarette smoking.

- Cancer of the breast—tends to be increased by obesity and high fat diets. A high level of alcohol consumption is currently being studied as a potential risk factor. Secondary prevention includes monthly breast self-exams and an annual medical examination.

- Cancer of the esophagus, mouth and tongue—cigarette, cigar and pipe smoking and chewing tobacco account for at least 90% of these cancers. Heavy alcohol intake has also been implicated in cancers of the esophagus.

- Cancer of the colon—this is the second most common form of cancer in the United States. Dietary factors account for about half of all colon cancers. The primary strategy for prevention is to eat enough dietary fiber (about 25–35 grams/day). An inverse relationship has also been found between colon cancer and physical activity.[3]

- Cancer of the cervix—it is extremely important to follow physician recommendations for regular Pap smear exams for secondary prevention.

- Cancer of the liver—heavy alcohol intake greatly increases the risk of liver cancer.

- Cancer of the skin—excessive sun exposure, particularly for fair skinned individuals, is the major risk factor. Malignant melanoma has been related to episodes of severe sunburn during the childhood years. Secondary prevention includes watching for changes in warts or moles and for small sores that don't heal.

No definite risk factors have been identified for cancer of the pancreas, stomach, prostate, or brain. Radiation exposure or chemotherapy may cause cancers of the blood (leukemias) and cancers of the lymph system.

3. Prevention of diabetes

NIDDM (non-insulin dependent diabetes mellitus, also known as Type II or adult onset diabetes) can often be managed or even avoided completely by implementing lifestyle modifications such as appropriate diet and exercise. A longitudinal epidemiologic study of adult men found that physical activity reduced the risk for developing diabetes, even when adjusted for obesity, hypertension and family history.[4] In addition, a diet high in complex carbohydrates that contains adequate fiber is important, as it seems to enhance glucose tolerance.

It should be noted that eating too much sugar is not the cause of diabetes. This misconception arises because diabetes is characterized by high levels of blood sugar (glucose). Excessive sugar consumption is indeed very dangerous for diabetics, who must curtail their sugar intake. However, sugar doesn't actually cause this disorder. Obesity appears to be the major risk factor in the development of adult onset diabetes, and sugar is not the major culprit in most cases of obesity. (Obesity is generally caused by physical inactivity and excessive calorie intake, with fat providing far more of the calories in the American diet than sugar.) While certain healthy lifestyle habits can help to prevent Type II diabetes, family history of the disease and age are uncontrollable risk factors.

4. Prevention of emphysema

Individuals suffering from emphysema, a chronic obstructive pulmonary disease (COPD), experience difficulty in breathing due to a narrowing of the bronchioles, or tubes carrying oxygen to the lungs, caused by physical damage to the lung tissues.

Over 90% of emphysema cases are caused by cigarette smoking. Unfortunately, once the disease process is in place, this condition does not reverse, although smoking cessation at any point is beneficial. Smoking destroys the cilia (small hairs that move mucous toward the mouth), distends and destroys the alveoli (air cells of the lungs), decreases lung elasticity, and leads to airway collapse and increased airway resistance. This process results in slow oxygen starvation with a great limitation in daily functional activities.

5. Prevention of cirrhosis

Cirrhosis results from three factors: repeated injury to liver cells, fatty change and death of liver cells, and the accumulation of fibrous scar tissue. These factors prevent adequate liver function. Excessive alcohol intake is directly responsible for about 75% of cirrhosis cases. After heavy scarring of the liver has occurred, cirrhosis is not reversible. Other kinds of liver injury, such as that caused by hepatitis, can also cause cirrhosis.

6. Prevention of osteoporosis and osteoarthritis

Osteoporosis (a condition of abnormally reduced bone density) can lead to easily fractured bones. Physical inactivity has repeatedly been shown to reduce skeletal bone mass and increase the likelihood of the development of osteoporosis.[5] Other modifiable risk factors are inadequate calcium intake, vitamin D deficiency, cigarette smoking, and consumption of more than two alcoholic drinks daily. Uncontrollable risk factors include being a female Caucasian or Asian, having a family history of this condition, having a small, delicate frame size, and experiencing early menopause.

Osteoarthritis, or degenerative joint disease, is the erosion of articular cartilage, usually as a result of mechanical joint stress or trauma. It can be minimized to some extent by maintaining an active lifestyle, avoiding obesity, and by protecting the joints from injury.

7. Prevention of back problems

Low back pain is a common problem, often estimated to afflict 80% of adults at some point in their lives. Back problems are the second leading cause of all office visits to primary care physicians (after colds).[6]

A majority of back problems are caused by weak or tight postural muscles, and chronic poor body mechanics in sitting, standing, lifting, exercising and sleeping activities. It is difficult to have proper body mechanics if the primary muscles affecting the spine are too tight or too weak. To prevent back pain and disability, strengthening the abdominals, spinal extensors, and scapular adductors, and stretching the spinal extensors, hip flexors, hamstrings and anterior chest muscles is helpful. Weight bearing exercise is necessary to keep the bone mineral content high and maintain bone density. Body awareness and proper lifting techniques need to be practiced. Since back problems frequently occur in overweight individuals, maintaining an appropriate weight is important.

8. Prevention of accidents

Most serious traumatic injuries are the result of automobile accidents. Seat belt use reduces the risk of sustaining a serious injury by about one-half and represents a choice to stay safe and healthy. Alcohol and/or drug intoxication is responsible for nearly one-half of all accidents. Don't drive or ride with anyone who is impaired.

How To Help Your Clients Promote their State of Wellness

As a personal fitness trainer, you should recommend the following six strategies for wellness maintenance and promotion to each client.

1. Exercise and remain moderately active

Remember that there are at least 50 well-documented benefits from physical activity as well as aerobic exercise, resistance training and flexibility work. Clients typically can list many negatives involved with exercising (sweat, need to shower, no time, etc.), but they can rarely list more than one or two benefits. Adherence will be better and motivation will be higher if clients understand how much there is to gain from an active lifestyle. According to one major study, fewer than 20% of U.S. adults engage in enough regular physical activity to receive any health benefits.[7]

According to a 1996 report from the Surgeon General on physical activity and health, "regular physical activity that is performed on most days of the week reduces the risk of developing or dying from some of the leading causes of illness and death in the United States." Regular physical activity improves health in the following ways:

– Reduces the risk of dying prematurely.

– Reduces the risk of dying from heart disease.

– Reduces the risk of developing diabetes.

– Reduces the risk of developing high blood pressure.

– Helps reduce blood pressure in people who already have high blood pressure.

– Reduces the risk of developing colon cancer.

- Reduces feelings of depression and anxiety.
- Reduces feelings of depression and anxiety.
- Helps control weight.
- Helps maintain healthy bones, muscles, and joints.
- Helps older adults become stronger and better able to move about without falling.
- Promotes psychological well-being.[88]

In addition, the Surgeon General's report makes three key points:

- People who are usually inactive can improve their health and well-being by becoming even moderately active on a regular basis.
- Physical activity need not be strenuous to achieve health benefits.
- Greater health benefits can be achieved by increasing the amount (duration, frequency, or intensity) of physical activity (see Chapter 4).

A moderate amount of physical activity can be achieved in a variety of ways, and doesn't necessarily have to be in the form of a formalized, structured exercise session to help reduce the risk of disease or premature death. Following are some examples of moderate amounts of activity:

- washing and waxing a car for 45–60 minutes
- washing windows or floors for 45–60 minutes
- gardening for 30–45 minutes
- wheeling self in wheelchair for 30–40 minutes
- walking 1¾ miles in 35 minutes (20 minute/mile)
- dancing fast (social) for 30 minutes
- pushing a stroller 1½ miles in 30 minutes
- raking leaves for 30 minutes
- shoveling snow for 15 minutes [88]

The Centers for Disease Control and Prevention and the American College of Sports Medicine have issued recommendations for physical activity that include the following:

- Every U.S. adult should accumulate 30 minutes or more of moderate-intensity physical activity on most, preferably all, days of the week.

– Physical activity can be accumulated in relatively short bouts.

– Adults who expend approximately 200 calories per day in moderate-intensity physical activity can expect many health benefits.

– Moderate physical activity is activity performed at an intensity equivalent to brisk walking at 3 to 4 mph for most healthy adults.

– Physical activity is closely related to, but distinct from, exercise and physical fitness. (Exercise is defined as "planned, structured, and repetitive bodily movement done to improve or maintain one or more components of physical fitness.")[89,86]

Physical activity and exercise are central ingredients of good health.

2. Eat a proper diet

The American Heart Association, the American Cancer Society, the National Cancer Institute, and the American Dietetic Association all basically agree on the dietary changes that individuals must make to reduce their risks of disease. Also, the Surgeon General's 1989 report confirmed the findings and recommendations of other organizations after a thorough review of the available evidence on diet and health. These guidelines include:

– Cut back on fat to 30% or less of total calories.

– Keep dietary cholesterol intake less than 300 mg/day.

– Limit sodium intake to no more than 2,400 mg/day.

– Decrease alcohol consumption.

– Increase carbohydrate consumption to 55–60% of total daily calories.

– Eat a variety of foods.

– Maintain an adequate calcium intake.

– Maintain a moderate protein intake from low fat sources.

3. Prevent obesity

Obesity is a condition characterized by excess body fat. It is associated with an increased incidence of hypertension, hyperlipidemia (excess fat or cholesterol in the blood), diabetes, degenerative arthritis, and certain cancers.[8] It increases the likelihood of hernias, hemorrhoids, gallbladder disease, varicose veins, and makes breathing more difficult. Excess weight makes everyday activities more problematic. Obese people are hospitalized more frequently than are people of average weight, and they have more surgical complications. Obesity is defined as a level of excess body fat that increases the risk of disease. Other characteristics of obesity include: having a body weight more than 20% above a desirable level, or having a percentage of body fat greater than 30% for women and greater than 20% for men.[9] Weight control is a two-fold process: weight reduction and weight maintenance, with weight maintenance being the most difficult aspect. There is some concern that the cycle of weight gain and weight loss (yo-yo dieting), particularly when unaccompanied by exercise, may lower the basal metabolic rate (BMR) and pose additional health risks.[10, 84]

4. **Stop smoking**

Cigarette smoking kills 307,000 people in the U.S. each year and is the leading cause of preventable death and disease according to the U.S. Surgeon General. Lung cancer and emphysema are perhaps the best known outcomes associated with smoking. However, heart disease is statistically the most serious problem resulting from smoking. The risk and frequency of heart attacks are greater in individuals who smoke, and increase according to the number of cigarettes smoked. In addition, the rate of heart attacks is lower among those who have given up smoking as compared with current smokers.[11] Smoking accelerates atherosclerosis, damages the lining of the arteries, increases total cholesterol, decreases HDL, and increases the stickiness of platelets, thereby increasing the risk of clotting. Smoking increases heart rate and blood pressure, causing the heart to require more oxygen. But, oxygen availability is compromised as carbon monoxide decreases the ability of the blood to carry oxygen.

The benefits of smoking cessation start almost immediately. Within two years, much of the risk of heart disease disappears, and within five to ten years, the risk is about the same as a non-smoker. Bronchitis and emphysema sufferers can expect an improvement in breathing almost at once. Nothing an individual can do, including diet and exercise, is as important as giving up smoking.

5. **Practice stress management**

Some examples of stress-related diseases, conditions and behavior are:

Cardiovascular system	Coronary artery disease Hypertension Stroke Rhythm disturbances of the heart
Muscular system	Tension headaches Muscle spasm backaches
Locomotor system	Rheumatoid arthritis Related inflammatory diseases of connective tissue
Respiratory and allergic disorders	Asthma Hay fever
Immunological disorders	Lowered resistance Autoimmune diseases
Gastrointestinal disturbances	Ulcer Irritable bowel syndrome Diarrhea Nausea and vomiting Ulcerative colitis
Genitourinary disturbances	Impotence Frigidity
Dermatological diseases	Eczema Neurodermatitis Acne
Other problems	Fatigue and lethargy Type A behavior Overeating and eating disorders Depression Insomnia

(From Beech, H. R., L. E. Burns and B. F. Sheffield, 1982. *A Behavioral Approach to the Management of Stress* (p.13) Wiley, New York, NY. Adapted by permission.)

Recent evidence suggests that hostility, cynicism, and chronic anger are the personality traits most closely linked to coronary heart disease risk.[12] The chronically angry, suspicious and mistrustful individual (as measured by objective tests) appears to be twice as likely to have coronary artery blockages. There are two major ways to break the stress/tension cycle: *physical* and *intellectual*.

Physical methods include but are not limited to: deep breathing techniques, stretching exercises, progressive muscle relaxation, biofeedback, counting backward, imagery and visualization, autogenic training, and meditation. These techniques all help to produce the "relaxation response" (decreased oxygen consumption, slowed metabolism, decreased resting heart rate and blood pressure, and increased alpha brain waves).

Intellectual methods include: improving communication skills, consciously choosing to change negative internal voices, and developing adaptive techniques for dealing with stressors (taking action against the stressors within one's control, and changing thoughts about the stressors beyond one's control).

6. Practice self-care

It is important to advocate self-responsibility to our clients. Individuals should appreciate and understand that they are in charge of their own health care management, working for prevention of diseases before they appear and for early detection and treatment of already existing illnesses. In general, healthy adults should have an annual physical and their blood pressure checked once a year (more if there is a family history of CHD); women over age 25 should have a Pap smear taken annually and should practice breast self-examination monthly; glaucoma tests should be implemented every few years after age 40 (especially if there is a family history); and dental checkups should be carried out annually.

The following are guidelines for prevention from the National Blue Cross/Blue Shield.

General Adult Screening Guidelines

Procedure	Recommendation
Pap smear for cervical cancer	First three tests to be done annually to ensure diagnostic accuracy. Every two to three years in sexually active women age 20–65. Every three years from age 66–75, regardless of sexual activity.
Fecal occult blood tests for colo-rectal cancer	Annually after age 50.
Sigmoidoscopy for colo-rectal cancer	Every three to five years after age 50. If family history of colon cancer in parent or sibling, air-contrast barium enema and sigmoidoscopy every three to five years after age 40.
Breast cancer screening	Monthly breast self-examination, with a breast exam performed yearly by a physician. Mammography should be done annually from age 40 on. Yearly mammograms may also be ordered in cases of fibrocystic disease.
Lung cancer screening	Screening not recommended.
Asymptomatic coronary artery disease screening	Screening with exercise stress testing generally not recommended for individuals with no symptoms who plan to exercise moderately. Those with symptoms or with disease, or older, higher risk clients planning to exercise vigorously should have a diagnostic exercise test.
Serum cholesterol screening	If less than 180 mg/dl, recheck every five years. If between 180–200, recheck within six months. For total cholesterol higher than 200, NCEP recommends a fasting lipid profile to determine LDL levels and subsequent treatment.
High blood pressure screening	Yearly; with family history every six months.
Diabetes screening	Every adult, starting at age 45, should be tested every three years. Those with high readings should repeat test on another day. Pregnant women do not need to be tested routinely if they are white, younger than age 25, of normal size and have no close family members with the disease.
Osteoporosis screening	Screening not recommended.
Visual acuity, glaucoma screening	Every two years and annually for those over 60.
Dental check-ups, gum disease	At a minimum, annually, however every six months is recommended.

IN SUMMARY

In this section, wellness was defined and steps for good health were outlined. Measures were considered for the prevention of coronary heart disease, cancer, diabetes, emphysema, cirrhosis, osteoporosis and osteoarthritis, back problems, and accidents. Six strategies were offered for helping clients practice prevention:

1. Exercise and remain moderately active
2. Eat a proper diet
3. Prevent obesity
4. Stop smoking
5. Practice stress management
6. Practice self-care

Chapter 2

The Initial Interview

The first session with a new client is simply a time to get acquainted. Using the effective communication skills discussed in Chapter 8, you will want to find out all you can about what your client wants and needs from you. Schedule an initial interview to acquire information, a physician's clearance, and a liability release. This must be done prior to fitness testing or exercise programming. This chapter describes forms used during the initial interview, and Appendix B has **sample forms** for reference.

The FitMarkers™ Questionnaire

The FitMarkers questionnaire is an assessment tool that can be used for clients who are non-physician referrals. This initial assessment can help you evaluate whether a client needs to be seen by a physician prior to further testing or the commencement of activity, or whether a client can safely participate in physical fitness assessments with gradual participation in exercise.

The FitMarkers questionnaire was developed along the same lines as the ParQ, as a "self evaluation" device. However, AFAA recommends that all clients (to help lower your risk of liability and maintain open channels to health care providers) receive medical clearance before beginning an exercise program. ACSM, on the other hand, recommends a physician referral based on age and number of cardiovascular risk factors.

During the initial interview, all five FitMarkers categories should be reviewed. An evaluation will be made based on the client's honest response to each question. The final determination will be categorized as either acceptable or unacceptable. If the client receives an unacceptable outcome, a referral should be made immediately to a physician and/or other health care professional(s) for medical clearance. If the client's outcome is acceptable, he/she should be able to safely complete further assessments and gradually progress into an exercise program.

The Medical History Form

The medical history form is an essential part of any client's entry procedure because it helps identify individuals at risk for cardiovascular, musculoskeletal, or other health problems. This health screening helps protect the client and is important for the personal fitness trainer (or club) from a legal and insurance perspective. The form and process should be carefully reviewed with your client, analyzing age, risk factors, possible symptoms of heart disease, pregnancy, orthopedic problems, medications, etc. If your client has risk factors requiring medical clearance, you will need to postpone the fitness assessment and/or exercise with the client until a personal physician has signed or stamped (in some cases a physician's signature stamp may be required in place of an actual signature), and returned the physician's clearance form to you. It is important to take appropriate action (e.g., refer for further evaluation or prescribe appropriate exercise program as deemed necessary) on any medical history information you obtain.

Steps for evaluating the medical history form

Step 1: Determine the client's age

Men age 40 or over and women age 50 or over should be cleared by their personal physicians.

Step 2: Analyze CHD risk factors

By definition, a health risk factor is any factor that increases the chance that an individual will develop a disease or condition. The more risk factors a person has, the greater the likelihood that he/she will have or develop a particular disease. Risk factors for CHD identified by the American College of Sports Medicine (ACSM) can be found in Chapter 1. The ACSM further defines a person's level of risk as follows:

Initial ACSM Risk Stratification

Low risk
Men <45 years old and women <55 years old who have no symptoms and zero or one risk factor

Moderate risk
Men >45 years old and women >55 years old, or those who have two or more risk factors

High risk
Individuals with one or more potential symptoms of coronary or metabolic disease, or with known cardiovascular, pulmonary, or metabolic disease

Step 3: Identify potential symptoms of coronary or metabolic disease

According to the ACSM[13], major symptoms that suggest cardiopulmonary or metabolic disease are:

- chest pain
- shortness of breath at rest or with mild exertion
- dizziness or fainting
- ankle swelling
- palpitations or irregular heartbeat
- cramping pains in legs or feet
- known heart murmur

A physician's clearance is recommended if:

1. There are two or more risk factors for CHD present
2. There are symptoms of cardiovascular, pulmonary, or metabolic disease
3. There is known cardiac, pulmonary or metabolic (including diabetes) disease
4. Your client is male and age 45 or over
5. Your client is female and age 55 or over

Step 4: Ascertain if your client is pregnant

The American College of Obstetricians and Gynecologists (ACOG) recommends that all pregnant clients be cleared for exercise by their physicians prior to starting an exercise program.[14]

Step 5: Other reasons to require a physician's clearance

Although there are no set guidelines from major organizations, it is advisable to request a physician's clearance for clients who have been recently hospitalized for any reason, who have chronic or acute muscle or joint injury, or who are on prescription medications.

If a client does not fall into any of the above categories, the client is then classed as apparently healthy and does not generally need medical clearance prior to fitness testing or exercise. In the event that a client has several risk factors, known disease, or medical complications or injuries, you may decide that your level of knowledge is insufficient to provide the safest monitoring and exercise programming for his/her condition. Know your limitations. It may be more prudent to recommend a cardiac rehabilitation facility or a physical therapist depending on the nature of the client's problem.

The Physician's Clearance Form

The physician's clearance form is important for several reasons. It helps reduce your liability and your client's risk, and it opens up communication between you and the physician. Always adhere to physician specified limitations.

Your client may need a diagnostic graded exercise stress test (GXT) prior to beginning an exercise program. This decision should be made by the physician.

The Exercise and Activity Quiz

The exercise and activity quiz gives you specific information about your client's activity level, exercise goals, past exercise history, and beliefs about exercise. It helps open the lines of communication between you and your client.

The Nutrition and Weight Profile

The nutrition and weight profile develops your client's awareness of his/her eating habits and helps educate him/her regarding healthy food choices. Relevant weight loss issues are raised, helping you understand your client better.

The Self-Assessment Quiz

The self-assessment quiz helps your client begin to understand wellness and the key benefits of wellness promotion. This quiz may be completed privately by the client and does not necessarily have to be returned to you. Its purpose is to educate.

Informed Consent

Informed consent should be obtained from every client prior to exercise testing or programming. Failure to warn clients about potential risks involved in exercise may be judged to be legally negligent. The informed consent form should explain in reasonable detail the exercise test and/or program, outline potential risks, dangers and discomforts, and describe the expected benefits. Clients should be advised of their responsibility to disclose all relevant information and ask any questions necessary to ensure a safe exercise experience. Check with an attorney for further advice.

Agreement and Release of Liability

The exercise waiver may be used for clients who refuse to obtain medical clearance or if you wish to secure an added potential measure of legal protection from suit. (It is strongly recommended that you insist on medical clearance for higher risk clients.) The use of such prospectively executed waivers, attempts to limit your liability for injuries sustained by your client as a result of the training and in some circumstances, even where the personal fitness trainer has proximately caused harm through his/her own negligent act or omission.

You should consult with legal counsel as to the enforcability of such documents and the requirements as to same state where services are to be provided.

Legal Considerations

- Always carry liability insurance. Professional groups, such as AFAA, offer reasonably priced group policies for fitness professionals.

- Always keep your certifications up-to-date. This is important not only to help establish your credibility as a professional in the event of a lawsuit, but to help ensure that you have continued your education and stayed current with fitness issues.

- Regularly update your clients' medical history forms and be aware of changes in their health status.

- Understand the limitations of your profession and activity. Unless you are a licensed physician, physical therapist, registered dietitian, chiropractor, massage therapist, social worker, psychotherapist, certified athletic trainer or other health care worker, you must avoid appearing to practice in these areas. Advice that you give to clients must not be construed as a diagnosis or a medical prescription. Also, you must refer clients to the appropriate health care provider and/or exercise setting when warranted by their health status.

- Document everything. Keep clear, appropriate and confidential records regarding your clients' health evaluations, fitness assessments, and session training logs. Document your clients' complaints, injuries and successes, as well as your responses.

- Plan for emergencies. Always know the location of the nearest telephone and how to activate the emergency medical system. Keep each client's emergency medical information with you for quick referencing during sessions. Always keep your CPR certification up-to-date.

- Your ultimate responsibility is to the safety of your client. Never leave a session unattended when you are being paid to work one-on-one. Be sure that your client's exercise equipment and workout area are safe, clean and in repair. Be certain that you have instructed your client in the proper use of all equipment.

- Stay up-to-date and follow exercise testing guidelines outlined by the ACSM. Do not attempt to administer maximal stress tests unless you have been specifically trained to do so. Refer specialized testing to physicians or exercise physiologists. When testing clients, always monitor the test properly and adhere to criteria for test termination as outlined by the ACSM.

■ Keep your instruction consistent with guidelines outlined by major organizations, such as ACSM, AFAA, NSCA, AHA, and the American Dietetic Association (ADA). Avoid contraindicated and controversial exercises; such exercises can put your client in harm's way and put you at risk of a lawsuit if a client is injured.

■ Be sure your clients' programs are appropriate for their health/fitness status, age, and ability to correctly carry out your instructions. This means selecting the appropriate intensity, frequency, duration and mode, as well as carefully instructing your clients as to the safe performance of the program.[15]

NOTE: For further reading on legal considerations, refer to Appendix A, under Legal Issues.

Case Study Practicum

A case study is a thorough evaluation of an individual: determining risk factors and health status, deciding whether or not to perform exercise testing, obtaining information from the fitness assessment and counseling sessions, and then formulating a plan for exercise programming.

To understand the process of critique, it is important to understand the key components of a case study. They are as follows:

■ Inclusion of month, day and year for each client visit

■ Description of client

■ Initial interview of client (including a review of and execution of all legal forms)

■ Outline of client's goals

■ Client assessments (objective measures used to collect data, e.g., health risk assessment, FitMarkers, fitness assessment, etc.)

■ Professional referrals given to client and their subsequent input

■ Interpretation and explanation of results from personal trainer and referral assessments

■ Development of exercise program based on interpretation of data and client's goals. Consider mode, frequency, intensity (including target heart rate range [THRR], and rate of perceived exertion [RPE] range), duration, and the rate of exercise progression over time

■ Implementation of program

■ Summary

When creating a case study leading to exercise prescription, you should consider the following questions:

1. What is your client's CHD risk factor profile, both primary and secondary?

2. Are there any other special limitations or medical conditions? What about the client's past medical history? Is the client taking any prescription medications which a health care provider has advised limits or contraindicates testing or exercise?

3. Do you need a physician's clearance prior to testing or exercising this client?

4. Should you perform a fitness assessment on this client or not? If so, what type of tests will you choose? (Decide for each test whether the benefit outweighs the risk and complete the informed consent process and forms for all such tests.) Consider cardiorespiratory, muscle strength and/or endurance, flexibility, postural, and body composition assessments. Be familiar with test endpoints and think about signs of fatigue that your client might exhibit.

5. Evaluate and interpret the results of the fitness assessment. Was everything normal?

6. Consider the client's interests, needs, goals, and level of motivation.

7. Have you formulated an exercise program based on all of the data collected? Have you considered mode, frequency, intensity (including target heart rate range [THRR], and rate of perceived exertion [RPE] range), duration, and the rate of exercise progression over time?

8. When will you retest your client?

9. What suggestions do you have for the client in terms of lifestyle modifications? What kind of counseling approach might work best with this client?

IN SUMMARY

In this section, initial steps for client health screening were outlined. This important process must take place prior to fitness assessment and/or exercise programming. The medical history form, physician's clearance, self-assessment quiz, exercise and activity quiz, nutrition and weight profile, informed consent, and exercise waiver were discussed. Relevant legal issues were covered in part and components of a case study were described.

Chapter 3

Fitness Assessment

After your client has filled out the appropriate forms and returned a signed physician's clearance form to you (if necessary), you are ready to perform a fitness assessment. Benefits of a fitness assessment include:

1. Establishing the client's current health status and providing you with baseline information. This information is valuable when developing your client's individualized exercise recommendations.

2. Utilizing this information for comparison later as the client progresses and improves.

3. Serving as a powerful educational and motivational tool, and increasing the likelihood of adherence.

4. When performed along with the prerequisite health screening, demonstrates your professional prudence and knowledge, which can be important if potential legal issues arise.

Limitations regarding fitness assessment include the fact that you are only predicting, or estimating, your client's fitness level. Avoid focusing on the absolute numerical values. What's important is to evaluate your client's progress; look at change over time. Use the fitness assessment to help your client focus on improvement.

Remember that prior to the actual exercise tests, your client needs to be informed about appropriate footwear and clothing and instructed to avoid drinking caffeinated or alcoholic beverages, smoking, or consuming a heavy meal for at least two hours before the fitness assessment. Nicotine, alcohol, a large meal and/or caffeine can all alter resting and exercising heart rate and blood pressure responses. Conversely, not eating anything for several hours prior to testing may cause a drop in blood sugar levels after the tests, leaving the client feeling dizzy, lightheaded or nauseous. In addition, have your client avoid exercising prior to the fitness assessment. Finally, if your client is ill or has recently had a viral infection, it is probably best to postpone the assessment.

Components of a Fitness Assessment

1. Assess resting heart rate and blood pressure (if possible)

2. Assess body composition (e.g., fatfolds, waist/hip ratio and girths)

3. Assess cardiorespiratory fitness (3-Minute Step Test or Rockport Walking Test)

4. Assess muscular strength and/or endurance (e.g., push-up test and crunch test)

5. Assess flexibility (e.g., Sit and Reach Test) and posture

6. Optional fitness assessment components

Step 1: Assess resting heart rate and blood pressure

Resting heart rate—A true resting heart rate is obtained first thing in the morning when the body is completely relaxed but conscious, before getting out of bed. Since even a true resting heart rate fluctuates, it's best to perform measurements on three consecutive days and take the average. In the fitness assessment setting, try to obtain as accurate a resting heart rate as possible by having the client sit quietly for 5–10 minutes prior to palpation. Heart rates fluctuate depending on the time of day, anxiety, stress, temperature, medication, smoking, eating and drinking (especially caffeine).

Resting heart rate may be palpated at the radial artery at the wrist for a full minute or for 30 seconds (multiply by two for the minute value). It is normal for some individuals (especially athletes) to have respiratory sinus arrhythmia at rest, meaning that the pulse speeds up during inhalation and slows during exhalation. For this reason, counting for 30 or 60 seconds at rest is more accurate than counting for 6, 10 or 15 seconds. It is also acceptable to palpate the pulse at the carotid artery at the side of the larynx on the neck, although it may not be as accurate if too much pressure is applied. Baroreceptors in the carotid artery detect pressure and may reflexively cause the heart rate to decrease. As a result, many professionals prefer that heart rate measurement be taken at the radial pulse.

An accurate resting heart rate is important for four reasons:

1. It is often used in the calculation of exercise target heart rate (Karvonen formula) for graded exercise tests and exercise prescription.

2. It can provide a baseline value for comparison as cardiovascular fitness improves (with training, an individual's resting heart rate usually decreases as his/her stroke volume increases).

3. Resting heart rate is sometimes used to assess cardiovascular fitness (printed norms are available[16]), although caution should be used in assessing a person's cardiovascular fitness solely on the basis of his/her resting heart rate.

4. Normal resting heart rates are usually regular (no palpitations), and are between 60–100 beats/minute. If your client's resting heart rate is over 100 bpm, under 60 bpm, or is irregular, a physician should be consulted. An exception is the aerobically trained athlete; it is not unusual for athletes to have resting heart rates as low as 40 bpm.

Resting blood pressure—Since high blood pressure, or hypertension, is one of the alterable risk factors for heart disease, and since an estimated one in four Americans (and, as a sub-group, one in three African Americans) has borderline or high blood pressure[17], routine measurement of resting blood pressure is very important. (However, check with the given state's laws and regulations as some states require that blood pressure only be taken by licensed health care providers.) It is recommended that all fitness professionals, particularly personal trainers, learn to monitor blood pressure. This becomes increasingly important should you decide to work with higher risk clients. During the fitness assessment, if your client has high resting blood pressure readings after three measurements, and has another risk factor (e.g., family history), then the client is classified as higher risk and further testing or exercise should be postponed until he/she is cleared by a physician.

Resting blood pressure can be affected by the same factors as resting heart rate (e.g., caffeine, stress, time of day). In addition, many clients become anxious about having their blood pressure measured, so relaxing quietly for 5–10 minutes prior to measurement may help.

Normal, or average, blood pressure is usually thought to be around 120/80 mm Hg. A person is not considered to have borderline hypertension until the values reach or exceed 140/90 mm Hg. ACSM defines diagnosed hypertension as systolic blood pressure >140, and/or diastolic blood pressure >90 mm Hg, on at least two separate occasions, or if the individual is on high blood pressure medication.[13] The top number, or higher value, is referred to as the systolic pressure, or the amount of pressure or force exerted against the arterial walls immediately after the heart has contracted. The bottom number or diastolic pressure, may be thought of as the "run off" force, or the amount of pressure still remaining against the arterial walls as the heart relaxes before the next contraction.

Measuring Blood Pressure—(*Note:* In some states, blood pressure may only be taken by a licensed health care provider. Always check with the given state's laws and regulations before taking such measurements.)

Blood pressure is measured with a stethoscope and a blood pressure cuff connected to a manometer (column or dial) from which the numerical values are read. (This device is called a sphygmomanometer.) Cuffs are available in child, adult, and large adult sizes. Size is important because too small a cuff on a large arm can result in a falsely elevated reading. Although this is no substitute for professional training in blood pressure measurement, generally, the procedure for taking blood pressure follows:

1. Place the cuff firmly around the upper arm with the lower edge approximately one inch above the bend in the elbow, or antecubital fossa. The middle of the bladder should be over the brachial artery on the inner part of the arm.

2. Place the bell of the stethoscope one inch below the cuff, directly over the brachial artery. (You may need to first palpate the brachial pulse at this site to be sure of placement.)

3. Inflate the cuff pressure to 200 mm Hg while listening through the stethoscope.

4. Slowly release the pressure at approximately two to three mm Hg per second. The point where the first rhythmic sound (called the first Korotkoff sound) is heard is the top number, or systolic pressure.

5. Continue to steadily release the pressure and note the point where the sound or pitch changes (fourth Korotkoff sound) and/or the point where the sound completely disappears (fifth Korotkoff sound). Usually the point where the sound disappears is considered to be the diastolic reading, although in some individuals the sound is occasionally heard all the way down to zero during exercise. In that case, the change in pitch signifies the diastolic pressure.

6. If the measurement needs to be repeated, be sure to wait approximately 60 seconds or more with the cuff completely deflated to allow circulation to return to normal.

    At rest, the client should have both feet flat on the floor and be in a relaxed sitting position with the arm supported. During aerobic exercise, it is normal for the systolic blood pressure (along with the heart rate) to increase with increasing work. The normal response of the diastolic blood pressure during exercise is to lower slightly (no more than 10 mm Hg), or to stay the same. However, if systolic blood pressure fails to increase, or if the diastolic blood pressure increases rapidly with increased work, then the exercise should be stopped and a physician should be consulted. Exercising blood pressure should be measured with the client's arm relaxed and not grasping a treadmill bar or cycle handlebar.

Note: These blood pressure measurement steps are illustrative only and should not be performed unless you have been trained in such measurement by a health care provider or qualified professional previously trained in such procedures. Performance of such measurement may be limited, by law, to licensed health care providers.

Step 2: Assess body composition

Although many clients may be interested in learning about their estimated percent body fat for cosmetic reasons, a primary reason for assessing body composition is to educate your client about the health risks involved with excessive body fat. It is well established that too much body fat is a health hazard and increases the risk of heart disease, diabetes, high blood pressure, some forms of cancer, low back pain, and other musculoskeletal problems. Body composition refers to the percentage of body weight that is fat and is based on the assumption that body weight can be divided into various components. Most equations use the two component model: fat mass and lean body mass (lean body mass is assumed to include, but is not limited to, muscles, bones, organs and internal fluids). The norms for body composition are based on equations that assume the densities for fat and lean body mass are the same for everyone. Therefore, the norms that you use to estimate your client's percent (%) body fat should ideally have been developed on a population with your client's same age, gender, race and physical activity level.

AFAA's recommendation for ideal % body fat for men is 12–17%, and for women is 18–22%. This is ideal, not average.

Your clients may find any or all of the following anthropometric assessments valuable:

 – Estimated % body fat
 – Body mass index
 – Waist to hip ratio
 – Girth measurements

Measuring estimated % body fat with the **skinfold caliper method**—The skinfold method of body composition assessment has been widely used and validated; when properly performed by experienced examiners it is relatively accurate. Calipers are used to measure the skin and subcutaneous fat thicknesses at selected sites (sites vary depending on the equations used). Calipers range in price from $15 to $350 with the more expensive models being more accurate and long lasting. The major disadvantage and source of error in the skinfold method is incorrect technique and/or lack of experience on the part of the examiner. It takes a great deal of time and practice as well as proper training to develop good technique. Always adhere conscientiously to the standardized guidelines below (from the Anthropometric Standardization Reference Manual, pp. 55-7018) to help ensure accuracy.

1. All measurements should be taken on the right side of the body.

2. Meticulously identify the site using anatomical landmarks.

3. Grasp the skinfold at the site to be measured with the thumb and forefinger of the left hand (the more subcutaneous fat a client has, the further apart your thumb and forefinger will need to be to grasp an adequate fatfold). Your left elbow should be angled up.

4. The grasp should be one centimeter (½ inch) above the site where the calipers will be placed to ensure that pressure from the fingers does not affect the measurement.

5. To be certain that only skin and fat have been grasped, you may, at some sites, ask your client to contract the underlying muscle while you continue holding the skinfold with your left hand. If you have inadvertently pinched muscle as well as fat, the muscle tissue will separate from the rest of the skinfold as the client contracts.

6. Holding the calipers in your right hand, take the measurement one centimeter (½ inch) below your left thumb and forefinger. The calipers should be held level and perpendicular to the direction of the skinfold. Release the jaws of the calipers completely (still holding the skinfold with your left hand) for no more than four seconds while you obtain the reading. (If the calipers remain pinching the skinfold for longer than four seconds, intracellular fluids will be forced out of the tissues and result in an inaccurate, lower value.)

7. A minimum of two measurements should be taken at each site. If your measurements vary by more than two millimeters, take a third or fourth measurement until you have obtained two measurements which vary by less than two millimeters. It is recommended that the measurements be taken in rotational order (e.g., triceps, suprailiac, thigh, then back to triceps, suprailiac, thigh), in order to avoid repeatedly compressing the tissues at the same consecutive site, resulting in smaller and smaller values.

Note: These skinfold measurement techniques and procedures are illustrative only. Personal training in such procedures is necessary prior to testing. Informed consent documents must include a description of such tests and the potential risks/benefits associated with testing.

Many population specific equations have been developed to predict body fat from skinfold measurements. Two of the most widely used equations appropriate for the general adult population (approximate ages 17–65) are those by Durnin and Womersley,[19] and those by Jackson and Pollock.[20] According to Lohman, the Durnin and Womersley equation yields slightly higher values.[18] Norms for the Jackson and Pollock equation can be found in Appendix C.

Standardized sites for women are:

Triceps—a vertical fold measured in the midline of the posterior arm over the triceps muscle. Anatomical landmarks are the lateral projection of the acromial process and the inferior border of the olecranon process with the elbow flexed at a 90° angle. A tape measure should be stretched between these two landmarks and the midpoint located on the lateral aspect of the arm. The actual site is at this level, only on the posterior aspect. During measurement, the right elbow should be extended and relaxed.

Suprailiac—a 45° angle diagonal fold immediately above the iliac crest along the anterior axillary line (this is different from the site used in the Durnin & Womersley protocol).

Thigh—a vertical fold in the midline of the anterior aspect of the thigh, midway between the inguinal crease (fold in the hip during hip flexion), and the proximal border of the patella. The body weight should be placed on the left leg so the right thigh is relaxed.

Standardized sites for men are:

Chest (pectoral)—a diagonal fold taken one half the distance between the anterior axillary line (underarm crease) and the nipple.

Abdomen—a vertical fold taken at a distance of two centimeters (one inch) to the right of the umbilicus. (This fold is horizontal in some other protocols.)

Thigh—same as for females (see above)

Calculating estimated % body fat:

1. Carefully measure the appropriate sites two to three times each, following the directions outlined above.

2. Find the average value for each site and then add all the sites together.

3. Using the norm tables titled "Percent Fat Estimations" in Appendix C, note where the sum of the skinfolds and your client's age intersect. This is the estimated % of body fat.

4. When counseling your client, emphasize improvement and progressive change of body fat levels over time. Avoid allowing clients to become fixated on a specific estimated number.

The Body Mass Index (BMI)—The body mass index was developed as a simple ratio of height to weight to use as an easy way to estimate body composition (and to classify degrees of obesity) for large groups. It is calculated by dividing body weight (in kilograms) by body height (in meters) squared (weight/height^2). You can also use the nomogram and the table for classification of obesity in Appendix C. Studies have shown the higher the body mass index, the greater the risk of negative health outcomes.[21] However, it should be noted that since the BMI does not take into account % body fat, it may not be as accurate at predicting risk for lean, athletic individuals.

Measuring waist to hip ratio—Where body fat is distributed is important. Studies have shown that when a greater amount of fat is stored in the abdominal area relative to the extremities, a person is at a higher risk for heart disease, diabetes and metabolic disorders. A method for assessing this risk is the waist to hip ratio—simply divide the waist circumference by the hip circumference.[9] If the ratio is greater than .95 for men or greater than .85 for women, the client is considered to be at higher risk and should be counseled about fat loss methods.

Taking girth (circumference) measurements—Clients are often interested in changes in their measurements as a result of an exercise program. Place the tape measure on the right side of the body for limb measurements; have your client stand erect but relaxed; take two measurements at each site (measurements should be within ¼ inch of each other); and avoid pulling the tape too tight or not tight enough. Consistency is key. (Special cloth tapes, known as Gulick tapes, are available to help standardize the tension.)

1. Abdominal—horizontal measure at level of umbilicus

2. Waist—horizontal measure taken at the level of the narrowest part of torso

3. Hips—maximum posterior protrusion of the buttocks

4. Thigh (proximal)—just below the fold of the buttocks

5. Upper arm—midway between the acromion and olecranon processes

6. Forearm—maximum circumference with elbow extended and palm supinated

7. Calf—maximum circumference between knee and ankle

Step 3: Assess cardiorespiratory fitness

Cardiorespiratory endurance, or aerobic capacity, is one of the most important components of fitness. Low levels of cardiorespiratory endurance have been associated with increased risk of premature death from all causes, most specifically from cardiovascular disease. In addition, greater aerobic fitness usually means that an individual is regularly active, and this has been linked with many health benefits.[22]

Aerobic or cardiorespiratory fitness is defined as the ability to perform repetitive, moderate to high intensity, large muscle movement for a prolonged period of time. VO_2 max (also known as maximal oxygen consumption or maximal oxygen uptake) is often considered to be one of the most important measures of aerobic fitness. It refers to the maximum amount of oxygen consumed and utilized by the body during an all out effort to exhaustion (such as during a maximal exercise test). It is assumed that this measurement represents the maximal capacity to resynthesize ATP aerobically. The more aerobically fit an individual is, the greater his/her ability to resynthesize ATP, and the higher her VO_2 max or ability to consume and process oxygen. VO_2 max is measured in either liters of O_2 consumed per minute (an absolute value), or in milliliters of O_2 consumed per kilograms of body weight per minute (a relative value).

Another important indicator of cardiorespiratory fitness is the anaerobic threshold, also known as the onset of blood lactate accumulation (OBLA). This is the point during exercise at which the work becomes so intense that muscle cells cannot produce the additional energy aerobically, and so begin to rely more and more on the anaerobic glycolytic pathway (lactic acid system) to produce ATP. At this level, lactic acid begins to accumulate and the so called lactate or anaerobic threshold is reached. When a person is aerobically fit, he/she can exercise at high levels of intensity without reaching this point, since the body, through training, adapts to consuming and utilizing large quantities of oxygen. Consequently, the anaerobic threshold, or level at which lactic acid begins to accumulate, is also quite high. Both VO_2 max and the anaerobic threshold increase with aerobic endurance training. Cardiorespiratory fitness can be evaluated with either maximal or submaximal exercise tests, and can be assessed either directly (with oxygen consumption equipment), or estimated (no oxygen consumption equipment is used).

Maximal exercise tests—These fall generally into two categories: diagnostic and functional. The purpose of a diagnostic exercise test (sometimes called a "stress" test or GXT) is to diagnose the presence and/or the extent of CHD in addition to evaluating ability to perform work (this is the type of test that a physician may recommend be performed on higher risk clients). The subject will be continuously monitored during exercise via a multi-lead ECG (electrocardiogram), and may or may not be using oxygen consumption equipment. This test usually takes place on a treadmill or cycle ergometer and the patient is pushed to achieve maximum work effort. By evaluating the ECG (especially at higher intensities), the physician or technologist can discern heart function abnormalities as well as cardiorespiratory endurance. Obviously, this kind of test should only be administered by highly trained personnel in a clinical setting. The purpose of a functional maximal exercise test is simply to assess cardiorespiratory fitness. It is often used to evaluate athletes and is important in research. VO_2 max is usually directly measured with oxygen consumption equipment as the subject exercises to exhaustion, most commonly on a treadmill or cycle.

The advantages of max tests include:

– The large amount of information gathered, including the actual measurement of a person's ability at high levels (however, there is still about a two percent range of error due to equipment and other factors) versus the estimated level obtained in submaximal testing.

– Specific cardiorespiratory responses to stress and high intensity enable the diagnosis of heart disease.

The disadvantages of max tests include:

– The need for special, expensive equipment and highly trained test administrators.

– Maximal testing is riskier than submaximal testing due to the potential for heart wave abnormalities at higher workloads.

– A high level of motivation on the part of the subject is necessary for exercise to exhaustion.

– All forms of testing are affected by the principle of specificity.

– Your clients will usually achieve higher test results when they are assessed performing an exercise with which they are familiar. For example, a cyclist will perform better on a cycle ergometer test than a client who never cycles, even though they may both be aerobically fit. However, on any piece of equipment it is still possible to assess a person's progress over time.

Another type of test requiring a maximal effort is the field test. The 1.5-mile run and the 12-minute run tests are widely used in college-type settings where it is necessary to test large groups of young athletes at once. Although inexpensive and easy to administer, these tests are higher risk due to their less supervised nature, and are not recommended for general population assessment. Norms are available.[29]

Submaximal exercise tests—There are many types of submaximal tests. Here the purpose is not to diagnose heart disease (ECGs are rarely used), but to assess the client's functional aerobic fitness, show improvement over time, and to help you prescribe an appropriate level of intensity. Submaximal tests may be used to predict or estimate VO_2 max, but the tests are concluded when a predetermined submaximal level has been reached (usually 85% of the estimated maximum heart rate), or when the subject has exercised for a specified time period (e.g., 3-Minute Step Test). The premise underlying submaximal testing is that the more fit an individual is, the lower his/her heart rate will be at any given level of intensity or workload.

The advantages of submaximal testing (as compared with maximal testing) include:

- less expensive
- less risky
- need less specialized equipment
- don't require as much training to administer

The major disadvantage of submaximal tests is:

- less accuracy if the purpose is to measure VO_2 max.

There are two basic types of submaximal tests: multi-stage (graded) and single stage (fixed load). A **multi-stage**, or **graded, submaximal exercise test** is based on two assumptions: 1) there is a linear relationship between VO_2 and heart rate, and 2) max heart rate can be predicted from the formula 220 - age = max heart rate. (In fact, this commonly used formula is accurate for only about 75% of the population. In the remaining 25%, max heart rate can vary from the formula by as much as 10–15 bpm, resulting in either an under or over prediction of max heart rate.[23]) Even with these limitations, a multi-stage submaximal test will provide you with valuable information about the client's cardiorespiratory responses and ability to perform work at various intensities, and therefore enable you to prescribe appropriate and accurate workloads during exercise sessions. Also, during follow-up re-tests, heart rate, RPE, and blood pressure responses to various workloads can be compared, allowing clients to see measured change in their cardiorespiratory fitness from the prescribed program.

Multi-stage tests can be performed on treadmills, cycle ergometers, or bench steps, and there are many different protocols (testing formats) available. At many commercial and corporate fitness facilities, the submaximal cycle ergometer test is the preferred form of aerobic fitness assessment. Advantages of the test are that the ergometer is easy to calibrate, relatively inexpensive and portable (as compared to a treadmill), nonintimidating to clients, and that heart rate and blood pressure are easier to assess during cycling exercise than during walking or running exercise. Also, in a multi-stage test, more information can be obtained than during a single-stage test. Disadvantages are that it may be difficult to maintain a constant speed or workload, localized muscle fatigue may limit performance, and the examiner needs specialized training to administer the test properly (i.e., at a university, or through ACSM or YMCA certification programs).

An alternative to the multi-stage test is the **single-stage (fixed load)** test. This test usually takes even less training to administer and requires less equipment. However, since there is only one stage, or workload, less information is obtained about your client. Heart rate, blood pressure, and RPE are usually not monitored during the actual exercise, which makes the test less useful for exercise prescription. Two types of submaximal fixed load tests are the 3-Minute Step Test and the Rockport 1-Mile Walking Test.

The **3-Minute Step Test**—The premise underlying the step test is that if a client has a low recovery heart rate one minute after stepping, he/she is in better physical condition and therefore has a higher VO_2 max and a higher level of aerobic fitness. The protocol for administering the 3-Minute Step Test follows:

1. Explain the purpose of the test to your client and describe the procedure. It is a good idea to suggest that clients refrain from conversation since talking, laughing, etc. may elevate their heart rate (although they must be encouraged to report any pain or discomfort). Static stretching of the gastrocnemius, hamstring and iliopsoas muscles may be advised; and a short practice session is allowed (two or three step cycles). There is no active warm-up.

2. Set the metronome at 96 bpm (24 step cycles per minute), and when the client begins stepping, start your timer or stopwatch. For this test, stepping must be performed on a 12-inch bench with a basic step pattern of up, up, down, down. The lead foot may change if necessary during the test (no continuous alternating lead). Have your client step for three full minutes, and let them know when one minute has passed, two minutes have passed, and when 10 seconds are remaining.

3. When the three minutes are up, remind the client to sit down immediately; within five seconds palpate the recovery heart rate (preferably on the radial artery at the wrist). Count the recovery heart rate for one full minute.

4. Use the minute value for the recovery heart rate and consult the norms appropriate for the client's age and sex on page 315. (Norms are also available that estimate VO_2 max based on recovery heart rate.[16])

The Rockport Walking Test—In 1986, the Rockport Walking Institute developed a test appropriate for the general population, including older and/or sedentary clients. The protocol follows:

1. Precede the test with a light warm-up consisting of rhythmic limbering and static stretching. Advise your client to stop at any time if he/she feels pain or discomfort, but that this test requires the most vigorous walk he/she can maintain for a mile.
2. The walking course needs to be smooth and flat, ideally a ¼ mile track. As your client walks, announce the time remaining with each lap.
3. After a mile has been completed, immediately palpate the pulse for 10 seconds (preferably on the radial artery). Allow your client to cool down.
4. Multiply the 10-second count by six and consult the norms for the client's age and sex in Appendix C (use both heart rate and completion time). Note that these norms are for men weighing 170 pounds and for women weighing 125 pounds. If your client weighs significantly more, then his/her aerobic fitness will be overpredicted; if he/she weighs significantly less, aerobic fitness will be underpredicted. Other factors that can influence the results are the client's level of motivation, ability to set a consistent pace, and level of body fat. (VO_2 max may be estimated using a generalized equation.[24])

When consulting clients about the results of cardiorespiratory testing, remember that VO_2 max numbers may have little meaning for them. They may be more interested in their increased stamina and enhanced ability to perform daily activities. Help them to see tangible proof of their improvement over time.

The Rockport Walking Treadmill Test—This test is very similar to the one outlined above. The protocol follows:

1. Precede the test with a warm-up consisting of static stretching and walking on the treadmill. Find the exact pace at which the client can walk vigorously for one mile.
2. Have the client walk at the established pace for one mile. Record the time.
3. Immediately palpate the pulse for 10 seconds and then allow the client to cool down.
4. Multiply the 10-second count by six and consult the norms for age and sex in Appendix C.

Note: All of the foregoing testing procedures must be preceded by the informed consent process, documented in writing, signed by the client and disclosing risks/benefits associated with such procedures. These testing procedures should never be performed by personal fitness trainers for diagnostic-type purposes, but rather, only for fitness assessment.

Step 4: Assess muscle strength and/or endurance

Muscle strength (the ability of a muscle or muscle group to exert maximal force for one repetition) and muscle endurance (the ability of a muscle or muscle group to exert submaximal force for several repetitions, or to hold a contraction for a sustained length of time) are both important components of fitness for your client's physical well-being. Without adequate muscle strength and endurance, clients are more likely to suffer from low back pain and/or poor posture, as well as other musculoskeletal problems. The development of muscle strength and endurance leads to an increase in lean body mass and an improvement in body composition, which in turn causes an elevation in resting metabolic rate. In addition, maintaining muscle strength and endurance is an important factor (especially for elderly clients) in performing everyday essential tasks adequately and without injury.

Assessing muscular strength—Muscle strength can be assessed either statically (isometrically) or dynamically (isotonically).

Static strength tests are most often performed on dynamometers. Dynamometers are available to assess hand grip strength and back and leg extensor strength, with the hand grip dynamometer being most widely used (keep in mind, this test does not measure a major muscle group and is therefore of limited predictive value). The procedure is simple: after adjusting the handgrip size for your client, have the client stand holding the dynamometer in one hand with the elbow flexed. Instruct him/her to exhale while squeezing as hard as possible (maximal voluntary contraction) for two to three seconds. Allow three trials for each hand and compare to the published norms.[25] Keep in mind that static strength tests are specific to the muscle group being tested and measure strength only at the particular angle at which the test is performed. Also, since clients tend to hold their breath and "bear down" (Valsalva maneuver) during isometric contractions, they must be instructed to exhale during exertion in order to prevent possible cardiovascular problems.

Muscular strength can also be assessed dynamically by the one-repetition maximum (1 RM) test. A frequently performed 1 RM test is the bench press, which assesses the strength of the pectoralis major, anterior deltoid, and triceps muscle groups. The client's maximum amount of strength for one repetition is found through trial and error. The procedure follows for the 1 RM Bench Press:

1. Have your client warm up by rhythmically limbering and statically stretching the muscle groups to be tested.

2. Familiarize the client with the equipment and have him/her start with a weight that can be comfortably lifted. Then progressively add weights until the weight can be lifted with proper form just one time (try to find the maximum amount within the first three attempts to avoid excessive fatigue). Allow the client to rest three to five minutes between trials.

3. After finding the 1 RM for the bench press, divide the 1 RM weight (in pounds) by the client's body weight (pounds) in order to apply the norms (see "Standard Values for Bench Press Strength..." in Appendix C).

Researchers have found that the 1 RM Bench Press (as well as the 1 RM Military Press), is the most valid measure of upper body strength.[26] (Norms also exist for the 1 RM Leg Press, which tests the muscle strength of the upper leg muscles.[26]) The test is relatively safe (especially when performed on a bench press machine), the subject's back is supported, the equipment is readily available in most fitness facilities, and the test is easy to administer. Disadvantages include the potential for injury that exists with any maximal effort, the fact that clients may perform the Valsalva maneuver, the lack of portability of the equipment, and the "intimidation factor" for clients unfamiliar with weights. In addition, some research indicates that the 1 RM test is not appropriate for beginners. To minimize a few of these disadvantages, some coaches recommend measuring a percentage of the client's 1 RM. For example, if your client can perform six but not seven repetitions of a bench press at 80 pounds, then he/she has a 6 RM of 80 pounds. Tables exist that allow you to then estimate the 1 RM value.[85]

Assessing muscle endurance—The most commonly performed tests for muscle endurance include the push-up test, the YMCA Dynamic Bench Press Test, the sit-up test, and the crunch test.

The **push-up test** measures upper body (pectoralis, anterior deltoid, and triceps) endurance, is easy to administer, and needs no special equipment. A disadvantage of the test is that performing even one push-up for deconditioned clients may require a maximal effort, and then the test no longer measures the ability to perform repeated contractions over time. The protocol is as follows:

1. Have your client assume the appropriate position: men on hands and toes (regular push-up), women on hands and knees (modified push-up). Instruct your client to breathe with each repetition and to repeat as many as possible with good form. Assure your client that he/she may stop if he feels any pain or discomfort.

2. Count the number of push-ups performed correctly. The spine should remain in proper alignment supported by the abdominals, with the neck continuing as a natural extension of the spine. The chest should come within three-inches of the floor (you may use your fist as a guide or use a three inch Nerf®-type or foam soft ball for clients to touch with each repetition).

3. The test is over when correct form can no longer be maintained or when your client is unable to complete another repetition. Norms are available in Appendix C.

The **Dynamic Bench Press Test**, developed by the YMCA, uses an external, standardized weight (barbell) of 35 pounds for women and 80 pounds for men. The barbell is lifted to a metronome count of 60 bpm (30 repetitions). The test is concluded when your client can no longer keep pace, begins to break form, or cannot complete another repetition. Published norms are available for ranking your client's upper body muscle endurance on the bench press.[16]

The **sit-up test** is also frequently used to assess the endurance of the trunk muscles. This test has been criticized because it involves not only the rectus abdominis but the iliopsoas muscle group. The client is asked to perform as many full sit-ups (elbows touching the knees) as possible in one minute while the feet are held in place by the personal fitness trainer. This test may aggravate existing low back pain and relies on an exercise (the full sit-up) that is not recommended for training. Norms are available.[16]

The **crunch test** has been recently developed as a safer modification of the sit-up test.[25] It is important to include some assessment of abdominal endurance when evaluating clients, since weak abdominal muscles with poor endurance have been linked with the development of low back pain. The protocol is as follows:

1. Have the client lie supine with knees comfortably bent, arms at sides with fingers pointing toward feet. The low back should remain on the floor at all times. Have the client curl up with head and shoulders off floor and slide hands a distance of six inches forward on the floor (you may use a ruler, a marked piece of tape, or your own hands as a guide). Allow one or two crunches for practice.

2. Begin the timer, and count the number of correctly performed crunches in one minute. Remind the client to exhale with each repetition.

3. You may compare the score with the norms for "Abdominal Crunch Test," listed by age and sex, in Appendix C.

Other tests for muscular fitness

Isokinetic testing—This form of assessment is used primarily in rehabilitation centers, and measures a muscle's tension throughout the full range of motion at a constant speed. It involves specialized, expensive equipment and is not widely available in commercial facilities.

Back tests—Since low back pain affects 80% of the population at some point, many tests have been developed to assess the strength, endurance and flexibility of the contributing muscle groups. A relatively safe test for assessing abdominal endurance was presented above. Other tests, such as the National Back Test and the Kraus-Weber test used by the Y's Way to a Healthy Back Program are available.[27] Both of these protocols use the one time performance of several exercises (e.g., both tests include a double leg raise with the feet held 10 inches off the floor and assess whether or not the client is able to keep the low back pressed to the floor for 10 seconds, thus measuring rectus abdominis endurance). The Kraus-Weber tests include prone spinal hyperextension for 10 seconds (measuring spinal erector endurance), and a one time standing toe touch. These tests are not without controversy and should only be administered by a qualified examiner, such as a physical therapist.

Anaerobic power tests—These tests measure a person's short term, power generating capabilities and are primarily used for performance athletes and for research purposes. Examples include the Sargent jump and reach test (measuring vertical jump), the standing broad jump test, running sprint tests, and cycling "sprint" or power tests (i.e., the Wingate power test). These tests are very intense and typically last only one minute or less; they are usually not appropriate for the general mixed population interested in health related fitness.

Note: As with other testing procedures, all strength related testing procedures should be preceded by a documented informed consent process.

Step 5: Assess flexibility and posture

Flexibility is defined as the range of motion possible around a joint. Like muscle strength and endurance, flexibility level is specific to each joint and its surrounding muscles. There is no single test that assesses total body flexibility. Flexibility assessment is important for clients; when range of motion is limited around a joint due to muscular tightness, that joint is more susceptible to injury. This is especially evident for proper functioning of the spine; tight erector spinae, hamstring, and iliopsoas muscles have all been implicated as possible causes of low back pain.

Also, ability to comfortably perform activities of daily living (such as bending over and picking up a piece of paper) is limited if the body is inflexible.

Flexibility is assessed directly by goniometers and flexometers. These tools actually measure the individual joint angle in degrees as the body part is moved through its range of motion.

In most commercial and corporate fitness settings, it is more common to assess flexibility indirectly, and perhaps the most widely performed assessment is the **Sit and Reach Test** used by the YMCA.[16] This trunk flexion test primarily measures the flexibility of the hamstring and erector spinae muscles, as well as the calf and upper back muscles (the flexibility of all of these groups is important for healthy low back functioning). Advantages of the test are that it is easy to administer, requires a minimum of equipment, and has widely validated norms. Disadvantages include the slight risk of injury due to the position required (seated unsupported forward flexion), and the fact that a person's score may be influenced by the length of his/her body segments, (for example, a long trunk and short legs). The procedure is as follows:

1. After explaining the purpose of the test to your client, have him/her actively warm up (if he/she is not already warm from the cardiorespiratory assessment) and perform some static stretching, particularly of the hamstrings, low back and calf muscles.

2. Instruct your client to remove his/her shoes and sit on the floor with knees straight (pressed to the floor), and the feet approximately 12 inches apart. The heels should be in contact with the sit and reach box with the ankles dorsiflexed. If no sit and reach box is available, a tape measure or yardstick may be used. The heels should be aligned at the 15-inch mark on the tape, with the zero end toward the body (the yardstick or tape can be secured to the floor with masking tape placed at a right angle to the 15-inch mark).

3. Have your client place his/her hands on top of each other with fingers aligned, and slowly exhale, stretch out, and touch the box, tape, or yardstick without bouncing. Allow your client to relax and then perform two more trials (total of three).

4. Your client's score is the best of the three trials and may be compared to the norms for his/her age and sex in Appendix C, listed under "Standard Values for Trunk Flexion."

Other flexibility tests

There are several other tests for specific joint range of motion and muscle flexibility, including:

Trunk extension ability—Have your client lie prone with hands on floor beneath shoulders. Attempt to push upper body up while maintaining hip contact with floor (passing flexibility of lumbar spine is with elbows fully extended and hips on floor). Use caution when performing this stretch: move slowly and stop immediately if there is any pain.

Hamstring flexibility—Have your client lie supine and lift one leg straight up while keeping the other pressed flat to the floor. Passing, or adequate hamstring flexibility, is the ability to lift the leg to a 90° angle, or to a vertical position, without straining. Assess both legs.

Hip flexor (iliopsoas) flexibility—Have your client lie supine. Clasp hands behind right knee and pull it in to the chest as far as possible. Keeping low back pressed to floor, extend the left leg and attempt to press back of left knee to floor. Adequate flexibility exists if the back of the knee and the low back can both be pressed to the floor simultaneously. Check both sides.

Quadriceps flexibility—Have your client lie prone with knees together. With right hand, gently pull right heel directly to middle of right buttock. Heel should comfortably touch buttocks for passing flexibility. Repeat on left side.

Calf (gastrocnemius and soleus) flexibility—Have your client stand with his/her back, hips and heels against a wall. Attempt to raise (dorsiflex) the right forefoot while keeping both knees straight. Passing, or adequate flexibility, is attained if the forefoot is able to be elevated by at least one inch. Repeat with the left forefoot.

Shoulder (deltoid, latissimus dorsi, triceps, rotator cuff muscles) flexibility—Have your client stand and raise left arm overhead and bend left elbow so that left hand points down the upper spine between the shoulder blades (hand should also be able to touch the opposite shoulder blade). Have your client bring his/her right arm behind the back, and bend the right elbow so the fingers point up the spine, between the scapulae. Good flexibility of the right shoulder exists if fingertips of both hands can touch. Change sides.

In addition to assessing muscle specific flexibility, these "tests" are valuable as a teaching tool, and they may all be used as stretches to enhance flexibility.

Postural screening

Many individuals have postural deviations that can predispose them to low back pain and/or other musculoskeletal problems. These assessments are simple, easy to administer, and help to develop client awareness.

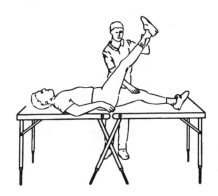

Fig. 3.1—Sit and Reach (demonstration of hamstring, erector spinae, calf and upper back flexibility)

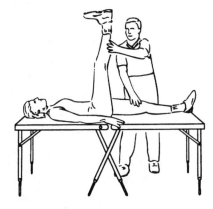

Fig. 3.2—Demonstration of hamstring flexibility

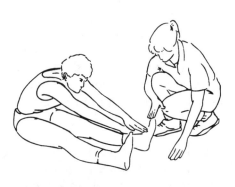

Fig. 3.3—Demonstration of tight hamstrings

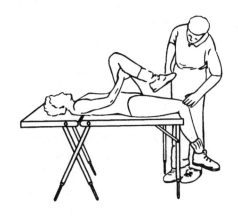

Fig. 3.4—Demonstration of hip flexor flexibility

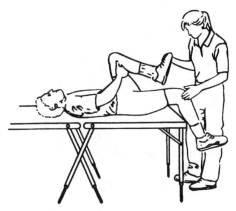

Fig. 3.5—Demonstration of tight hip flexor

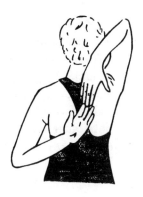

Fig. 3.6—Demonstration of shoulder flexibility

Lordosis (swayback) assessment—Have your client stand in normal alignment with shoulders and hips against a wall, feet hip width apart, heels one inch from wall. Have client relax, breathe normally, and avoid consciously pressing low back to wall. Normal lumbar curvature exists if you can slide your palm between client's lower back and the wall without forcing. If a large gap (greater than one palm depth), is found, your client may have a tendency towards lordosis, and should strengthen the abdominals and stretch the iliopsoas and erector spinae muscles. (Also observe client's bony anatomy: the anterior superior iliac spine of the ilium should not be in front of [anterior to] the pubic bone.)

Kyphosis and forward head assessment—Have your client stand normally and observe posture from the side. There is a tendency toward kyphosis if the upper back appears hunched or slouched forward and the shoulders appear rounded. "Forward head" may or may not accompany this position. Forward head stance is indicated if the ears are not in line with the shoulders and/or the chin juts forward. If these tendencies exist, clients will need to strengthen scapular adductors (mid-trapezius and rhomboids), and stretch shoulder horizontal adductors (pectoralis major and anterior deltoids).

Hip and shoulder height discrepancies—If a significant hip and/or shoulder height discrepancy exists, your client may have scoliosis, or lateral curvature of the spine. If this condition is accompanied by back pain or discomfort, further evaluation by a physician is needed. Also, it may be inappropriate for clients with scoliosis to participate in high- impact activities, such as running or high-impact aerobics, due to increased risk of injury. (Note: Such clients must be referred to a health care professional for clearance for a particular activity before that activity is recommended to them.)

To **measure hip height/leg length discrepancy**, have your client remove his/her shoes and stand normally with feet a comfortable hip width apart. Place one end of tape measure on iliac crest (top of hip bone), and bring other end down outside of leg to the floor, past the lateral malleolus (outside ankle bone). Measure both sides, making sure to be consistent from right to left sides in terms of tape placement.

To **measure shoulder height discrepancy**, tape a large piece of paper at shoulder height on wall. Have your client stand normally against wall with shoulders pressed against paper, hips back, and heels one inch from wall. Place a level clipboard or notebook on right shoulder and draw a horizontal line on the paper. Repeat with left shoulder, making sure to be consistent in terms of clipboard placement. Measure distance from each horizontal line to floor with tape measure.

For both hip and shoulder height assessments, a discrepancy of ¼ inch or greater between right and left sides may suggest a misalignment, or possibly scoliosis. (Misalignments may be due to many causes, including improper footwear, muscle imbalances, or habitually carrying a handbag, baby, small child, etc., on one side.)

Postural screening abnormalities that are noted by you should be discussed with your client along with recommendations that your client seek assessment and advice by a health care professional.

Step 6: Optional fitness assessment components

Other assessment options, depending on your client, skill, equipment, and knowledge base, might include a stress management/coping strategy questionnaire, three-day dietary recall, lung function tests, and cholesterol testing.

Lung function can be assessed with a portable spirometer. Two values are usually obtained: forced vital capacity (FVC), the total volume of air that can be moved through the lungs in one breath from full inhalation to a maximum exhalation, and forced expiratory volume (FEV1), the percentage of the vital capacity that can be expired in one second (indicating the speed that the air can be moved through the lungs). In average healthy people, approximately 85% of the vital capacity can be expired in one second. Less than 70% FEV1 would indicate some type of airway obstruction difficulty (such as with emphysema or bronchial asthma).

Several types of cholesterol tests are available. Some facilities offer their clients relatively inexpensive, fasting blood lipid profiles performed by an outside laboratory. This is the most accurate test, as it requires the client to fast for 12 hours, and the blood is returned to the lab for LDL, HDL, triglyceride and total cholesterol analysis. Some facilities have on-site equipment for cholesterol testing, such as Reflotron, Vision, or Kodak DT-60™. Although the initial purchase of these machines is costly and the person operating the machine needs some training, this type of basic cholesterol screening can be a valuable adjunct to other forms of fitness and wellness assessment. The test is quick, no fasting is required, immediate results are available, and the results are relatively accurate. Disadvantages include the fact that only total cholesterol is assessed, lengthy calibration and quality control procedures are essential to ensure accuracy, and some states require that only phlebotomists or other medical personnel may use finger sticks to draw blood due to the possibility of contamination from blood borne pathogens if correct procedures are not followed.

Finally, consider developing "functional" fitness tests that are specific to your individual client's goals. Assessing physiological parameters, such as heart rate and RPE after climbing a flight of stairs or taking a routine walk with the dog, can be a very practical way to measure change over time. When you choose activities that the client performs regularly and in which the client wants improvement, "functional" fitness tests can provide yet another way to validate your client's exercise program and enhance adherence.

Putting It All Together

Procedure	Materials needed

I. The Initial Interview

Tell the client about yourself, and ask what she/he is looking for. Perform a health screening:

a. Have client fill out the FitMarkers questionnaire or medical history form.	FitMarkers questionnaire or medical history form.
b. Review forms and determine need for a signed physician's clearance form prior to testing and/or exercise.	Physician's clearance form.
c. Give client the physician's clearance form if necessary.	
d. Have client read and/or read to him/her and sign informed consent (including delineated risks/benefits) and answer questions.	Informed consent.
e. Give client other forms to fill out (depending on client).	Self-assessment quiz, exercise and activity quiz, nutrition and weight profile.
f. Discuss payment and business arrangements.	
g. Give information about clothing, footwear, abstaining from caffeine, smoking, etc. prior to fitness test.	

II. Fitness Assessment (If a signed physician's clearance is necessary, postpone fitness assessment until form is returned.)

a. Assess resting values. - Take a 30 or 60-second resting HR. - Take a resting blood pressure.	Stopwatch. BP cuff and stethoscope.
b. Assess body composition. - Estimate % body fat with skinfold calipers, and/or calculate body mass index, and/or take tape measurements for comparison at retests. - Assess waist to hip ratio.	Calipers, calculator, tape measure, norms, nomogram for BMI.
c. Assess cardiorespiratory fitness. - Perform either the 3-Minute Step Test or the Rockport 1-Mile Walking Test.	Stopwatch, 12-inch bench and metronome, OR smooth, flat ¼ mile track and stopwatch.
d. Assess muscle strength and/or endurance. - Options include: 1 RM tests, push-up test or crunch test.	Machines, mat, tape, norms.
e. Assess flexibility and posture. - Options include: Sit and Reach Test, muscle specific tests, posture tests.	Sit and reach box or tape measure or yardstick and masking tape, mat, paper taped to wall.
f. Perform other optional assessments.	

III. Interpretation and Goal Setting Session

Depending on time factors, you may or may not decide to present the results of the fitness assessment at the same session as the actual testing. Results should always be presented in a positive manner. No matter how your client scored on a particular test, encourage him/her not to focus on a specific numerical score, but instead to focus on the fact that if he/she adheres to an exercise program, there will be change and improvement over time. Review the five components of fitness and the importance of reducing risk factors, and encourage a larger view of health and wellness. Educate and motivate!

Help your client to have a reasonable expectation about his/her exercise program and its expected results. Both preparing for a realistic experience and establishing achievable goals have been proven to help with exercise adherence and long lasting behavior change. Help the client define specific, focused goals that are measurable and attainable. Short-term goals of four weeks or so are more effective than long-term goals (e.g., lose 50 pounds). At the end of each goal period, reevaluate client progress and give appropriate feedback. During the goal setting session, create a "game plan" as to exactly how your client will reach his/her goal and be specific with exercise dates, times, places, attire and dietary modifications (a goal setting form is provided in Appendix B). Specify the date for fitness test reassessment. Allow approximately three months for measurable benefits, such as decreased resting heart rate, increased aerobic capacity, and decreased % body fat. Be sure to encourage the less quantifiable internal reinforcements of progress, such as enhanced self-esteem, decreased stress and increased energy. Consider using a behavioral contract to enhance compliance (see Appendix B).

Based on client feedback during this session, the next task is to formulate an appropriate exercise prescription.

IN SUMMARY

In this chapter, benefits and limitations of fitness assessment were discussed. The following components of the fitness assessment were covered: 1) Assess resting values; 2) Assess body composition; 3) Assess cardiorespiratory fitness; 4) Assess muscle strength and/or endurance; 5) Assess flexibility and posture; and 6) Optional assessment components. An interpretation and goal setting session was discussed and recommended for increased client education, motivation and adherence to exercise. Adherence to informed consent procedures and documentation was also stressed.

Chapter

4

Cardiorespiratory Programming

Cardiorespiratory fitness is defined as the ability to perform repetitive, moderate to high intensity, large muscle movement for a prolonged period of time. Many health benefits and training adaptations have been associated with aerobic fitness.

Benefits of Cardiorespiratory Fitness Include:		
■ stronger heart	■ increased stroke volume	■ decreased resting HR
■ lowered BP	■ increased cardiac output	■ increased caloric expenditure
■ increased HDLs	■ improved cholesterol ratio	■ increased metabolism
■ stronger bones	■ decreased stress and depression	■ increased endurance, stamina and energy
■ improved sleep		
■ decreased body fat	■ improved immune function	■ increased ability to metabolize fat
■ increased ability to perform work with less fatigue (increased functional ability)	■ improved glucose tolerance and insulin sensitivity	
	■ improved quality of life	

The American College of Sports Medicine has published guidelines and position statements for health enhancement, and for the development of cardiorespiratory fitness.[13,28] In general, the guidelines for health enhancement are at a slightly lower threshold than those for cardiorespiratory fitness. In other words, individuals may exercise at lower levels (40–50% of VO_2 max) and still see reductions in health risk factors. This is especially important for very deconditioned or inactive clients. For these clients, adopting a moderately active lifestyle may significantly improve their health and may be a more attainable goal than achieving a very high level of fitness. As clients become more fit, Position Stand recommendations should be followed in order to see significant changes in VO_2 max and body composition. The Position Stand is summarized below:

ACSM Position Stand	
Frequency	3 to 5 days/week
Intensity	50–85% HRR or VO_2 max or 65-90% of maximum HR
Duration	20 to 60 minutes of continuous or intermittent aerobic activity
Mode	Any activity that uses large muscle groups, can be maintained continuously, and is rhythmical and aerobic in nature
Progression	Depends on functional capacity, health status, age, and client preferences and goals; three stages: initial, improvement and maintenance

In addition, ACSM recommends minimal thresholds of 300 kcal per exercise session performed three days per week, or 200 kcal per session performed four days per week. To achieve optimal physical activity levels, the goal is to bring the weekly expenditure closer to 2000 kcal as health and fitness progresses.

To improve the cardiorespiratory system, overload must occur. Manipulating frequency, intensity, duration and mode are all ways to overload and cause improvement to the cardiorespiratory system. Increases in VO_2 max (the maximal ability of the body to consume, transport and utilize oxygen) may range from 5% to 30%.

All exercise sessions should be preceded by a warm-up. According to AFAA guidelines, the 8–12 minute warm-up should consist of a balanced combination of rhythmic limbering (i.e., large, full-body movements that increase body temperature and increase blood flow to the heart and muscles), and static stretching (held, sustained preparatory stretches lasting 8–10 seconds for major muscle groups). Aerobic activity should be followed by a post-aerobic cool-down phase, a three- to five-minute period (or longer if needed) of gradually decreasing intensity that helps prevent blood pooling in the extremities and reduces feelings of dizziness. Stretches may be repeated and held for 10–20 seconds each.

Frequency

The ACSM recommends a frequency of three to five days per week. For weight reduction purposes, four to five days per week are better than three. Research shows that exercising more than five days per week has little effect on VO_2 max, and increases the risk of injury and burn-out. Extremely deconditioned clients may benefit from several short daily exercise sessions. High-impact activities are associated with higher risk of injury and probably should be avoided on a daily basis by non-conditioned individuals.

Intensity

Intensity is the most complex of the training variables. It is interrelated with duration; together, intensity and duration determine the total calorie cost of an exercise session.

The total amount of work performed is one of the most significant factors in improving cardiorespiratory fitness. Improvement is similar for low-intensity, long-duration activities versus high-intensity, short-duration activities if the total energy costs of the activities are equal. However, high-intensity exercise carries a higher risk of cardiovascular complications, orthopedic injuries, and decreased adherence. Low- to moderate-intensity training programs with longer durations are recommended for most adults.[28] In addition, due to the large number of sedentary adults and the associated increased health costs and mortality, the ACSM, the Centers for Disease Control and the U.S. Surgeon General's Report state that even moderate levels of physical activity may offer substantial health benefits.[86,88] In other words, any type of activity is better than none at all.

The ACSM recommends an intensity of 50–85% of heart rate reserve (HRR) max (or VO_2 max) for improvements in both health and fitness, and includes guidelines for very deconditioned individuals of 40–50% of heart rate reserve max.

Prescribing exercise intensity

Methods for figuring how hard your client should exercise are nearly the same as those used to assess intensity while exercising. Methods of prescribing intensity include:

1. HR methods: percentage of HR max and the Karvonen (HRR) method

2. Rate of perceived exertion (RPE scale or Borg scale)

3. Using METS to establish the proper workload

1. Heart rate methods

Prescribing and measuring intensity by taking a pulse is very common and convenient. However, this method has some limitations, including: the effect of medications (may decrease or increase the HR); the fact that both HR methods are based on the formula 220 - age = max HR (accurate for only about 75% of the population[23]); the effect of the pressor response (HR elevated due to upper body exercise, but oxygen consumption and calorie expenditure are not consistent with HR); and the initial difficulty teaching clients to take an accurate pulse.

1. Heart rate methods

– Percentage of maximal heart rate

This method is very simple and is used in the ubiquitous target heart rate charts found in most clubs. It will yield a more conservative target heart rate than the Karvonen formula. There are two steps:

1. 220 - age = estimated max HR
2. estimated max HR x percentage (e.g., 70%) = target HR

– Karvonen formula (heart rate reserve method)

This method, which factors in resting heart rate, yields training ranges that correspond more closely to percentage of functional aerobic capacity ranges. (If a client performs a graded maximal exercise test, VO_2 max can be measured and a training range can be determined as a percentage of VO_2 max. This is not practical for most clients.) The Karvonen formula has four steps:

1. 220 - age = estimated max HR
2. estimated max HR - resting HR = HR reserve (HRR)
3. HRR x percentage (e.g., 70%) = percent of HRR
4. percent of HRR + resting HR = target HR

In both of the above methods only one target HR is obtained. Since clients need a target HR range (e.g., 70%–80%), the calculation should be repeated for the second percentage as well (e.g., 80%).

– How Do You Select the Appropriate Percentages?

This is an arbitrary decision based on at least four factors:

1. client's risk factors and/or any orthopedic limitations
2. client's level of fitness (estimated during the fitness assessment)
3. client's goals
4. client's level of motivation

Finally, since both HR methods yield a target HR in beats per minute (e.g., 160 bpm), a final step should be added for clients. Divide the target HR by six to get a 10-second value (AFAA recommends taking the pulse for 10 seconds at the radial artery).

2. Rate of perceived exertion (RPE) method

This method is valuable for assessing and prescribing intensity for several reasons, including: it may be used even if clients are taking HR altering medications; it helps clients to "listen to their bodies;" it provides an accurate gauge of approaching fatigue; and it is a widely validated, reproducible tool for monitoring intensity.[29] RPE can be used in conjunction with the heart rate method.

RPE (Borg) Scale		Revised RPE Scale	
6	No exertion at all	0	No exertion at all
7	Very, very light	0.5	Very, very weak
8		1	Very weak
9	Very light	2	Weak
10		3	Moderate
11	Light	4	Somewhat strong
12		5	Strong
13	Somewhat hard	6	
14		7	Very strong
15	Hard	8	
16		9	
17	Very hard	10	Extremely strong
18		*	Maximal
19	Extremely hard		
20	Maximal Exertion		

© Gunnar Borg, 1985, 1994.
For correct usage of the scale see Borg's Perceived Exertion and Pain Scales, Champaign, IL. Human Kinetics, 1998.

Using the original Borg scale, a rate of 12–13 approximates 50% of HRR and a rate of 16 approximates 85% of HRR. Therefore, the ACSM recommends that clients exercise within an RPE range of 12–16 (meaning, to the clients, that the intensity subjectively feels somewhat hard to hard). On the revised scale, this would be between four and six. Clients can be given a range (e.g., 12–14) as part of their prescription. Most people will need instruction to help them understand how to use the RPE scale; extremely unfit or inactive clients may need two to three sessions before they use the scale properly.

3. Using METS to establish the proper workload

A MET (metabolic equivalent) is a unit of energy expenditure often used by physiologists and cardiologists. Most people, on a pound per pound basis, consume approximately the same amount of oxygen at rest ($VO_2 \approx 3.5$ ml of O_2/Kg of BW/min[1] with BW=body weight). This resting oxygen uptake value is equivalent to one MET. In other words, having an energy expenditure of one MET means that an individual is expending only a resting level of energy (calories). If a person exercises at a five MET level of energy expenditure, that means he/she is consuming five times more oxygen and calories than at rest. (5 x 3.5 ml/Kg/minute would equal 17.5 ml of O_2 consumed per Kg of body weight per minute.) Therefore, 10 METS equals 10 times resting, and so on.

If your client performed a graded exercise stress test, MET values, which are useful when deciding what intensity is appropriate, can be obtained. For example, if your client reached maximum, a percentage (e.g., 50–85%) of the maximal MET level can be used. If your client had symptoms of heart disease at a certain MET level, then exercise programming would obviously take place below that MET level. Also, many cardiologists specify the MET levels at which they want their patients to exercise. The energy cost (MET level) of most daily activities and exercises is known (see below). Equations exist that allow you to calculate the MET levels for various running, walking, cycling and stepping workloads.[13]

HR and RPE prescriptions stay relatively constant as your client's fitness level improves; with training adaptation, a given workload feels easier (and HR decreases), so your client has to work harder to stay in his/her target HR range. MET levels (workloads) need to be increased as aerobic endurance progresses.

Energy Expenditure in METS of Various Activities		
	Mean	**Range**
Archery	3.9	3–4
Backpacking	—	5–11
Badminton	5.8	4–9+
Basketball		
Game play	8.3	7–12+
Non-game	—	3–9
Billiards	2.5	—
Bowling	—	2–4
Boxing		
In-ring	13.3	—
Sparring	8.3	—
Canoeing, rowing and kayaking	—	3–8
Conditioning exercise	—	3–8+
Climbing hills	7.2	5–10+
Cricket	5.2	4–8
Croquet	3.5	—

Cycling		
To work or for pleasure	——	3–8+
10 mph	7.0	——
Dancing (social, square, tap)	——	3–8
Dancing (aerobic)	——	6–9
Fencing	——	6–10+
Field hockey	8.0	——
Fishing		
From shore	3.7	2–4
Wading in stream	——	5–6
Football (touch)	7.9	6–10
Golf		
Power cart	——	2–3
Walking (carrying bag or pulling cart)	5.1	4–7
Handball	——	8–12+
Hiking (cross-country)	——	3–7
Horseback riding		
Galloping	8.2	——
Trotting	6.6	——
Walking	2.4	——
Horseshoe pitching	——	2–3
Hunting (bow or gun)		
Small game (walking, carrying light load)	——	3–7
Big game (dragging carcass, walking)	——	3–14
Judo	13.5	——
Mountain climbing	——	5–10+
Music playing	——	2–3
Paddleball, racquetball	9	8–12
Rope jumping	11	——
60–80 skips/minute	9	——
120–140 skips/minute	——	11–12
Running (see below)		
Sailing	——	2–5
Scuba diving	——	5–10
Shuffleboard	——	2–3
Skating, ice and roller	——	5–8
Skiing, snow		
Downhill	——	5–8
Cross-country	——	6–12+
Skiing, water	——	5–7
Sledding, tobogganing	——	4–8
Snowshoeing	9.9	7–14
Squash	——	8–12+

Soccer	——	5–12+
Stair climbing	——	4–8
Swimming	——	4–8+
Table tennis	4.1	3–5
Tennis	6.5	4–9+
Volleyball	——	3–6
Walking (see below)		

From ACSM. 1995. *Guidelines for Exercise Testing and Prescription* (5th ed.). Media, PA: Williams and Wilkins.

Selected MET Levels of Walking and Running on the Treadmill

Elevations	0%	2%	4%	6%	8%	10%	12%
Speed (MPH) Walking							
2.0	2.5	3.1	3.6	4.2	4.7	5.3	5.8
2.5	2.9	3.6	4.3	5.0	5.7	6.3	7.0
3.0	3.3	4.1	4.9	5.8	6.6	7.4	8.3
3.5	3.7	4.6	5.6	6.6	7.5	8.5	9.5
4.0	4.1	5.2	6.3	7.4	8.5	9.6	10.7
Speed (MPH) Running							
5.0	8.7	9.4	10.0	10.7	11.4	12.1	12.8
5.5	9.4	10.1	10.9	11.7	12.5	13.2	14.0
6.0	10.2	11.0	11.8	12.7	13.5	14.3	15.2
6.5	11.1	12.0	12.9	13.8	14.6	15.6	
7.0	11.7	12.7	13.6	14.6	15.6		
7.5	12.5	13.5	14.6	15.6			
8.0	13.3	14.4	15.5				

(calculations made by author, Mary Yoke, 1996)

Methods of assessing intensity (finding out if your client is working at an appropriate level) include:

1. Measuring HR to determine if your client is in his/her target HR range.

2. Asking your client to rate his/her perceived exertion.

3. Using the talk test (or breathlessness test). Your client should be able to talk and breathe comfortably during aerobic exercise. A possible exception might be the highly fit and motivated client who is performing sprint-type work above the anaerobic threshold.

Duration

The ACSM recommends 20 to 60 minutes of continuous aerobic activity. This does not include warm-up and cool-down. Duration is inversely related to intensity—the lower the intensity, the longer the duration may be. For very deconditioned clients, several low intensity, short duration (<10 minutes) sessions may be preferable. Duration can then be gradually increased as your client adapts to training.

Mode

Mode refers to the type of activity that is used for cardiorespiratory improvement. The greatest improvement in VO_2 max results from repetitive, rhythmical use of the large muscle groups for a prolonged period of time (>20 minutes). Activities that are considered to be aerobic include, but are not limited to: walking, running, cycling, swimming, stepping, aerobic dance, rowing and cross-country skiing. Some activities are useful for developing aerobic endurance if the individual has the skill to perform them continuously. These include such activities as: skating, jumping rope, tennis, racquetball and basketball.

Since high-impact activities (e.g., running, jumping rope, and high-impact aerobic dance) have been linked with high risk of injuries, low-impact activities are recommended for beginners and those vulnerable to orthopedic problems. Also, cross-training helps to prevent boredom and may reduce the risk of injury.

It is important to find a type of activity (or several activities) that your client enjoys and will do. This is essential for long-term adherence and behavior change.

Progression

There are three stages of progression depending on your client's functional capacity, health status, age, needs and goals. These are the initial, improvement and maintenance stages.

- Initial conditioning stage—This stage is especially critical for the less fit and/or inactive client. The foundation is laid for long-term increased physical activity and healthy lifestyle changes, with the main purpose of establishing an exercise habit. For these clients in particular, it is important not to be too aggressive in programming, to find activities they enjoy, minimize injury and soreness, and encourage a sense of inner satisfaction with the exercise process. Set them up for success with realistic goals and an appropriate initial exercise prescription. This stage should include light muscular endurance exercises and low-level aerobic activities (40–60% of HR reserve). Duration may begin with 12–15 minutes or less and gradually progress. Three non-consecutive days per week are desirable.[13] This stage typically lasts four to six weeks for the less fit client.

■ Improvement stage—In this stage, progression is more rapid. Frequency, intensity, duration and mode may be manipulated to cause progressive, yet gradual overload to the cardiorespiratory system. Many trainers systematically increase one or more of these factors every two to three weeks depending on the client's ability to adapt.

■ Maintenance stage—When a client reaches his/her fitness goals, maintenance and adherence can become goals in themselves. Cross-training and variety in programming are two possible strategies to help with compliance.

Cardiorespiratory Training Systems

There are several options in training methods for aerobic fitness, including:

■ Continuous training

■ Interval training

■ Fartlek training

■ Super circuit training

■ Cross-training

Continuous training

Often called long, slow, distance training (LSD), this type of program involves exercising at the same workload for a prolonged period of time (20–60 minutes), without a rest interval. For example, Mr. C. walks on the treadmill at 4 mph, 3% grade continuously for 25 minutes. This protocol is safe and easy to teach to clients. Beginners may prefer this type of training. The major disadvantage is that it may become boring.

Interval training

Interval training may be used for all levels of participants. It involves repeated bouts of harder work interspersed with periods of easier work (or, occasionally, rest periods). For less fit clients on the treadmill, this may mean three minutes of "easy" work at 3 mph and 0% grade, then one minute of "hard" work at 3.5 mph and 0% grade. This might be repeated five times for a total of 20 minutes. The client could be encouraged to work at a "12" on the RPE scale during the easy bout, and at a "14" on the RPE scale during the hard bout.

This type of training can be utilized all the way up the fitness ladder. For extremely fit clients, the program may consist of four minutes of running at 9 mph, alternated with one minute of relief at 8 mph, and so on. Advantages of this type of training are that the total amount of work performed may be greater than continuous training, clients may find it less boring and thus be more likely to adhere, and it is easy to systematically cause progressive overload.

Fartlek training

Similar to interval training (but less structured), Fartlek, or speed play training, is very demanding and is therefore more appropriate for fit, low-risk, motivated clients. It involves free form, non-systematic alternations between high speed, high intensity, anaerobic work and low intensity, relief type periods.

Super circuit training

Super circuit, or aerobic circuit training, alternates aerobic exercise stations with resistance exercise stations. For example, three minutes on the treadmill, then one minute leg press, three minutes stairclimber, one minute lunges, three minutes cycle, one minute lat pull-down, three minutes rower, one minute bench press, etc. Advantages of this type of format are that it helps eliminate boredom, can work equally well for class-type settings as well as one-on-one, and allows a large amount of total work in a short period of time. Clients need to be familiar with the exercises and equipment that will be used, as they will need to move quickly from one station to the next.

Cross-training

Aerobic cross-training can be applied in several different ways:

1. Using a variety of cardiorespiratory equipment within one workout, e.g., ten minutes on the cycle, ten minutes on the treadmill, ten minutes on the stairclimber.

2. Using a variety of equipment (or modalities) throughout the week, e.g., Monday: run 30 minutes; Wednesday: cycle 40 minutes; Friday: cross-country ski 25 minutes; Saturday: play singles tennis for one hour.

3. Periodizing cross-training involves the use of different modalities across large blocks of time or seasons, e.g., summer: emphasize swimming and training for windsurfing; fall: versa-climber, outdoor rock-climbing and tennis; winter: cross-country and downhill skiing; spring: running and canoeing.

Advantages of cross-training are decreased risk of injury and reduced risk of burn-out due to boredom.

IN SUMMARY

In this section, the benefits of cardiorespiratory fitness are listed and the ACSM Guidelines and Position Stand for health enhancement and cardiorespiratory fitness were discussed. Specifics of intensity programming were covered, including heart rate methods, perceived exertion, and METS. Frequency, duration, mode and progression were discussed, as well as several cardiorespiratory training systems.

Chapter

5

Kinesiology Review

Knowing kinesiological and anatomical terms makes it much easier to talk about the body, discuss positions and movements for exercise, and communicate with other health fitness professionals. In addition, in order to plan effective exercises for your clients, it is essential to know which muscles perform which joint actions.

Joint Actions

(These definitions assume that movement takes place from the anatomical position.)

> *Flexion*—movement that shortens the angle between two bones. Most flexion movements are forward movements. Major exception is knee flexion.

> *Extension*—movement that increases the angle between two bones. Most extension movements are backward movements. Major exception is knee extension.

> *Lateral Flexion*—bending of the spine to the side.

> *Adduction*—movement toward the midline of the body.

> *Abduction*—movement away from the midline of the body.

> *Horizontal Flexion/Horizontal Adduction*—movement toward the midline of the body in the horizontal plane.

> *Horizontal Extension/Horizontal Abduction*—movement away from the midline of the body in the horizontal plane.

> *Rotation*—medial or lateral movement around an axis.

> *Circumduction*—movement in which an extremity describes a 360° circle.

Supination—the lateral rotation of the forearm, bringing the palm of the hand upward. In this position, the radius and ulna are parallel.

Pronation—medial rotation of the forearm, with the palm in a downward position so the radius lies diagonally across the ulna.

Eversion—rotation of the foot with the sole turned outward (sometimes referred to as pronation).

Inversion—rotation of the foot with the sole turned inward (sometimes referred to as supination).

Dorsiflexion—movement that brings the top of the foot toward the shin.

Plantarflexion—movement that brings the sole of the foot downward (pointing the toes).

Depression—downward movement of the shoulder girdle.

Elevation—upward movement of the shoulder girdle.

Scapular adduction (also known as retraction)—backward movement of the shoulder girdle with scapulae pulled toward the midline.

Scapular abduction (also known as protraction)—forward movement of the shoulder girdle with scapulae pulled away from the midline.

Scapular upward rotation—rotation (or upward turning) of the scapula in the frontal plane with the glenoid fossa facing upward.

Scapular downward rotation—return from upward rotation.

Scapular upward tilt—a turning of the scapula on its frontal-horizontal axis so that the superior border turns slightly forward-downward and the inferior border moves slightly backward-upward (and away from the rib cage).

Reduction of upward tilt—return movement from upward tilt.

Line of pull—the direction of the muscle from its origin to its insertion. The line of pull across a joint will determine the function(s) of the muscle.

Planes

Planes geometrically bisect the body and describe bodily movements. (Movements take place alongside or next to the planes.) There are an infinite number of parallel planes to each plane listed below.

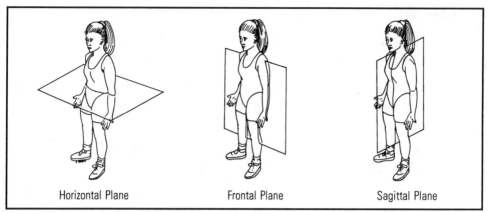

| Horizontal Plane | Frontal Plane | Sagittal Plane |

Fig. 2.1

Horizontal plane—(sometimes called transverse) divides the body into upper and lower portions.

Frontal plane—(sometimes called the coronal) divides the body into front and back. Abduction and adduction occur within the frontal plane.

Sagittal—(occasionally called the medial) divides the body into right and left portions. Flexion and extension occur within the sagittal plane.

Positions and Directional Terms

Anterior—to the front

Posterior—to the back

Lateral—away from the midline

Medial—toward the midline

Superior—above

Inferior—below

Superficial—on or near the surface of the body

Deep—further from the surface of the body

Proximal—closer to the trunk

Distal—further from the trunk

Supine—lying on the spine (on the back)

Prone—lying face down

Joint Movers

Agonist—prime mover, or the contracting muscle that is responsible for the movement that you see.

Antagonist—the muscle that works in opposition to the prime mover and reflexively elongates to allow the agonist to contract and move the joint.

Assistor—the muscle that assists in performing a movement, but is not a prime mover. Sometimes called a secondary mover.

Stabilizer—the muscle that maintains a static or isometric contraction to anchor or support the movement of the primary mover.

Synergist—textbooks disagree on the definition of a synergist. Some describe it as a stabilizer; some describe it as an assistor. The muscle is contracting synergistically along with the prime mover in some way.

Muscle Contractions

When muscles "work," or develop force or tension, they are said to contract. However, this implies that the muscles shorten. Muscles sometimes shorten when they work, but they can also lengthen or even stay the same length and still produce tension. There are three main types of muscle actions:

Isometric—a held, static muscle action where there is no change in the joint angle or muscle length. Strength gains that result from isometric contractions are joint angle specific. A disadvantage of an isometric contraction is the tendency for breath holding (Valsalva maneuver) leading to a rise in blood pressure, which may be dangerous for some clients.

Isotonic or dynamic—muscle actions that are not held, but that have movement. In most exercise settings, this is the most common type of action. Muscle tension varies throughout the range of motion depending on mechanical factors. There are two types:

Concentric—shortening contraction of a muscle as it develops tension against a resistance (often called a positive contraction).

Eccentric—lengthening action of a muscle as it develops tension against a resistance (often called a negative contraction).

Isokinetic—muscle actions performed on special equipment where speed is controlled, and any force applied against the machine results in an equal reaction force. This type of contraction is considered by many practitioners to be very safe; consequently, this equipment is most often found in the clinical rehabilitation setting.

Muscle and Joint Attachments

Ligament—band of fibrous tissue that connects bone to bone and provides joint stability. Ligaments are non-elastic; once stretched, they remain stretched.

Tendon—dense, fibrous connective tissue that forms the end of a muscle and attaches the muscle to bone.

Fascia—fibrous connective tissue that forms sheaths for individual muscles.

Cartilage—white, semi-opaque, fibrous connective tissue that cushions the joints and prevents wear on articular (joint) surfaces.

Synovial membrane—a thin tissue surrounding most movable joints that secretes synovial fluid. This fluid provides nourishment, lubrication and hydrostatic cushioning.

Bursae—liquid-filled membranes that protect soft tissues as they pass by bony projections.

Muscle Terminology

Smooth muscle—a type of muscle tissue that is present in many organs (e.g., intestines), and is generally not under voluntary control.

Cardiac muscle—an entire structure of interconnected cardiac fibers that contracts involuntarily as a unit.

Skeletal muscle (striated muscle)—muscle tissue that causes joint movement and is under voluntary control. Skeletal muscles can have several types of fiber arrangements:

Fusiform muscle—fibers are arranged parallel to the line of pull, usually in a spindle shape, tapering at each end (e.g., biceps brachialis).

Longitudinal muscle—a long strap-like muscle with parallel fibers (e.g., rectus abdominus).

Fan shaped or triangular muscle—a flat muscle whose fibers radiate from a narrow end to a broad end (e.g., pectoralis major).

Pennate muscle—densely packed muscle fibers are arranged oblique to the line of pull in a feather-like arrangement. May be unipennate (e.g., tibialis posterior), bipennate (e.g., retus femoris), or multipennate (e.g., deltoid).

IN SUMMARY

In this section, the benefits of cardiorespiratory fitness are listed and the ACSM Guidelines and Position Stand for health enhancement and cardiorespiratory fitness were discussed. Specifics of intensity programming were covered, including heart rate methods, perceived exertion, and METS. Frequency, duration, mode and progression were discussed, as well as several cardiorespiratory training systems.

Shoulder Joint Muscles and Their Actions

	Flexion	Extension	Abduction	Adduction	Internal Rotation	External Rotation	Horizontal Flexion	Horizontal Extension
Anterior deltoid	P.M.		Asst.		Asst.		P.M.	
Medial deltoid			P.M.					P.M.
Posterior deltoid		Asst.				Asst.		P.M.
Supraspinatus			P.M.					
Pectoralis major, clavicular	P.M.		Asst.*		Asst.		P.M.	
Pectoralis major, sternal		P.M		P.M	Asst.		P.M	
Coracobrachialis	Asst.			Asst.*	Asst.*	Asst.+	P.M.	
Subscapularis	Asst.^		Asst.^	Asst.*	P.M.		Asst.	
Latissimus dorsi		P.M.		P.M.	Asst.			Asst.
Teres major		P.M.		P.M.	P.M.			Asst.
Infraspinatus						P.M.		P.M.
Teres minor						P.M.		P.M.
Biceps, long head			Asst.					
Biceps, short head	Asst.			Asst.	Asst.		Asst.	
Triceps, long head		Asst.		Asst.				

* Indicated action takes place only when arm is above the horizontal.

+ Indicated action takes place only from a position of rotation to the neutral point.

^ Assistant actions vary with joint position and activity of synergistic muscles.

P.M. = Prime Mover; Asst. = Assistant Mover

Shoulder Girdle Muscles and Their Actions

	Elevation	Depression	Abduction	Adduction	Upward Rotation	Downward Flexion
Subclavius		Asst.				
Pectoralis minor		P.M.	P.M.			P.M.
Serratus anterior			P.M.		P.M.	
Trapezius I	P.M.					
Trapezius II	P.M.			Asst.	P.M.	
Trapezius III				P.M.		
Trapezius IV		P.M.		Asst.	P.M.	
Levator scapulae	P.M.					
Rhomboids	P.M.			P.M.		P.M.

NOTE: Movements of the arm on the trunk involve the cooperative actions of the shoulder joint and the shoulder girdle, as well as the attached muscles. Pure isolation of these muscles is often not possible. For instance, joint actions in this area are frequently caused by muscles acting as a force couple (equal parallel forces pulling in opposite directions), e.g., trapezius II and serratus anterior act together to cause upward rotation.

Elbow and Radioulnar Joint Muscles and Their Actions

	Flexion	Extension	Pronation	Supination
Biceps brachii	P.M.			Asst.
Brachialis	P.M.			
Brachioradialis	P.M.		Asst.*	Asst.*
Pronator teres	Asst.		Asst.	
Pronator quadratus			P.M.	
Triceps brachii		P.M.		
Anconeus		Asst.		
Supinator				P.M.
Flexor carpi radialis	Asst.		Asst.	
Flexor carpi ulnaris	Asst.			
Palmaris longus	Asst.			
Extensor carpi radialis longus		Asst.		Asst.
Extensor carpi radialis brevis		Asst.		
Extensor carpi ulnaris		Asst.		
Flexor digitorum superficialis	Asst.			
Extensor digitorum		Asst.		
Extensor digiti minimi		Asst.		
Extensor pollicis longus				Asst.
Abductor pollicis longus				Asst.

*To the mid position

Knee Joint Muscles and Their Actions

	Flexion	Extension	Inward Rotation	Outward Rotation
Biceps femoris	P.M.		P.M.	
Semitendinosus	P.M.		P.M.	
Semimembranosus	P.M.			P.M.
Rectus femoris		P.M.		
Vastus lateralis		P.M.		
Vastus intermedius		P.M.		
Vastus medialis		P.M.		
Sartorius	Asst.		Asst.	
Gracilis	Asst.		Asst.	
Popliteus*	Asst.		P.M.	
Gastrocnemius	Asst.			
Plantaris	Asst.			

* "Unlocks" the knee at the start of knee flexion

Hip Joint Muscles and Their Actions

	Flexion	Extension	Abduction	Adduction	Inward Rotation	Outward Flexion
Psoas	P.M.		Asst.			Asst.
Iliacus	P.M.		Asst.			Asst.
Sartorius	Asst.		Asst.			Asst.
Rectus femoris	P.M.		Asst.			
Pectineus	P.M.			P.M.	Asst.	
Gluteus maximus		P.M.	Asst.*	Asst.+		P.M.
Gluteus minimus	Asst.~	Asst.*	Asst.		P.M.	Asst.*
Gluteus medius	Asst.~	Asst.*	P.M.		Asst.~	Asst.*
Tensor fasciae latae	Asst.		Asst.		Asst.	
Biceps femoris		P.M.				Asst.
Semitendinosus		P.M.			Asst.	
Semimembranosus		P.M.			Asst.	
Gracilis	Asst.			P.M.	Asst.	
Adductor longus	Asst.			P.M.	Asst.	
Adductor brevis	Asst.			P.M.	Asst.	
Adductor magnus	Asst.*	Asst.+		P.M.	Asst.	
The six outward rotators #						P.M.

Piriformis, Obturator internus, Obturator externus, Quadratus femoris, Gemellus superior, Gemellus inferior
* Upper fibers   + Lower fibers   ~ Anterior fibers   • Posterior fibers

Ankle Joint Muscles and Their Actions

Extrinsic Muscles	Dorsiflexion	Plantarflexion	Inversion	Eversion
Tibialis anterior	P.M.		P.M.	
Extensor digitorum longus	P.M.			P.M.
Peroneus tertius	P.M.			P.M.
Extensor hallucis longus	Asst.		Asst.	
Gastrocnemius		P.M.		
Plantaris		Asst.		
Soleus		P.M.		
Peroneus longus		Asst.		P.M.
Peroneus brevis		Asst.		P.M.
Flexor digitorum longus		Asst.	Asst.	
Flexor hallucis longus		Asst.	Asst.	
Tibialis posterior		Asst.	P.M.	

(From Rasch, P. and Burke, R. 1989. *Kinesiology* (7th ed.), Baltimore, MD: Williams & Wilkins)

THE HUMAN SKELETON—ANTERIOR VIEW

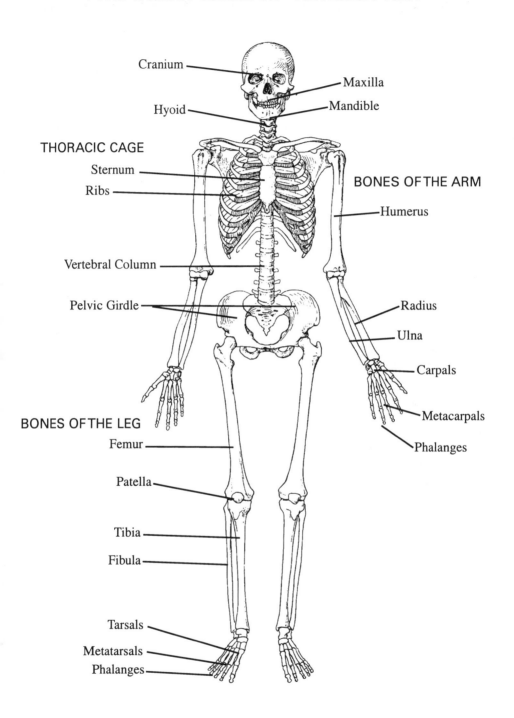

Cranium

Maxilla

Hyoid

Mandible

THORACIC CAGE

Sternum

Ribs

BONES OF THE ARM

Humerus

Vertebral Column

Pelvic Girdle

Radius

Ulna

Carpals

Metacarpals

Phalanges

BONES OF THE LEG

Femur

Patella

Tibia

Fibula

Tarsals

Metatarsals

Phalanges

THE HUMAN SKELETON—POSTERIOR VIEW

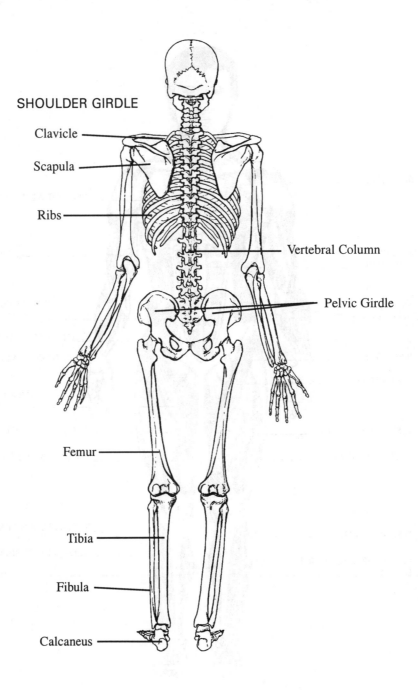

SHOULDER GIRDLE

Clavicle

Scapula

Ribs

Vertebral Column

Pelvic Girdle

Femur

Tibia

Fibula

Calcaneus

MUSCULAR SYSTEM—ANTERIOR VIEW

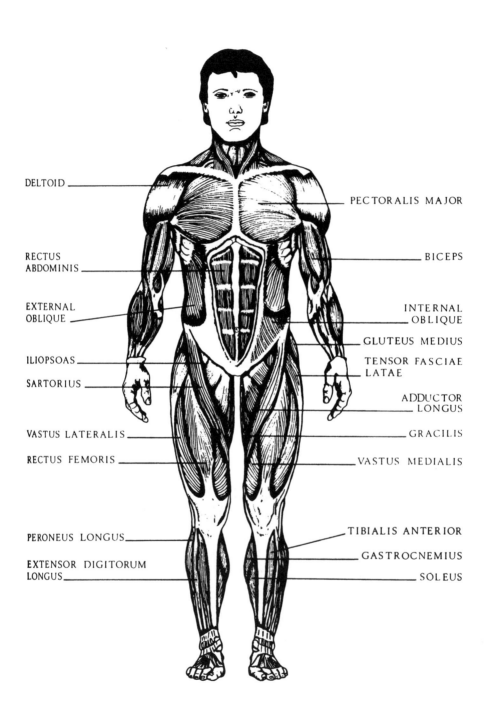

DELTOID

RECTUS
ABDOMINIS

EXTERNAL
OBLIQUE

ILIOPSOAS

SARTORIUS

VASTUS LATERALIS

RECTUS FEMORIS

PERONEUS LONGUS

EXTENSOR DIGITORUM
LONGUS

PECTORALIS MAJOR

BICEPS

INTERNAL
OBLIQUE

GLUTEUS MEDIUS

TENSOR FASCIAE
LATAE

ADDUCTOR
LONGUS

GRACILIS

VASTUS MEDIALIS

TIBIALIS ANTERIOR

GASTROCNEMIUS

SOLEUS

MUSCULAR SYSTEM—POSTERIOR VIEW

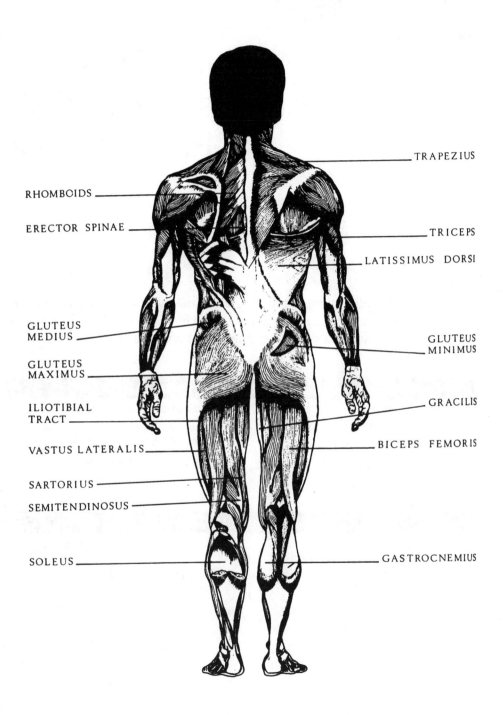

RHOMBOIDS

ERECTOR SPINAE

GLUTEUS MEDIUS

GLUTEUS MAXIMUS

ILIOTIBIAL TRACT

VASTUS LATERALIS

SARTORIUS

SEMITENDINOSUS

SOLEUS

TRAPEZIUS

TRICEPS

LATISSIMUS DORSI

GLUTEUS MINIMUS

GRACILIS

BICEPS FEMORIS

GASTROCNEMIUS

Chapter

6

Muscular Strength, Endurance and Flexibility Programming

Muscular strength and endurance (muscular fitness) are components of fitness (along with cardiorespiratory fitness, flexibility and appropriate body composition) that are important for overall health and well-being.

Benefits of Muscle Strength and Endurance Include:

- increased capacity to perform work (increased functional ability)
- increased bone mass
- decreased risk of injury
- increased motor performance
- increased strength of connective tissue (muscles, tendons, ligaments)
- increased fat-free mass resulting in increased metabolism

Circuit Weight Training May Also Result In:

- modest improvements in cardiorespiratory fitness (about 5%)
- improved glucose tolerance
- modest reductions in blood pressure
- improved blood lipid profiles

Muscle Structure

Muscle fibers

Skeletal muscles contain bundles of muscle fibers. Each muscle fiber is a muscle cell. Muscle fibers contain myofibrils which have a basic functional unit known as a sarcomere. Within each sarcomere are thin myofilaments that cause muscle action. These are the proteins actin and myosin. Each muscle fiber is innervated by a single motor nerve; that nerve and the other muscle fibers attached to it make up the motor unit.

The Huxley sliding filament theory is the most widely accepted theory explaining muscle shortening. Cross-bridges, or myosin heads, are thought to attach to specialized sites along the actin filaments, causing the myosin and actin to slide past each other in opposite directions. ATP provides the energy needed for the cross-bridges to attach.

There are two major fiber types: fast twitch (FT) fibers, and slow twitch (ST) fibers. Most skeletal muscles have both types of fibers. However, the percentages of FT and ST fibers are not the same in all muscles of the body, or from person to person. ST (Type I or slow oxidative) fibers are slow to fatigue and have a high level of aerobic endurance. FT fibers have poor aerobic endurance. FT fibers have two broad subdivisions: fast twitch a (also known as Type IIa or fast oxidative glycolytic), and fast twitch b (also known as Type IIb or fast glycolytic). Both types of fast twitch fibers tend to produce ATP anaerobically. Fast twitch IIa fibers are used in short duration, high intensity activities, and fatigue quickly. Fast twitch IIb fibers are not used often and are stimulated by extremely high intensity, maximum strength, explosive type events.

Fibers are generally recruited for exercise according to the size of the motor unit, with the smaller motor units being utilized first. FT fibers have very large motor units when compared to ST fibers. Therefore, FT fibers are the last to be recruited since they are more difficult to stimulate. Recruitment order is ST, and then FT (fast twitch IIa and then fast twitch IIb). FT fibers are stimulated whenever a large amount of total force is needed, e.g., very heavy weights or high velocity type movements.

Proprioceptors

Proprioceptors are sensory organs found in muscles, joints and tendons that give information to the brain concerning movement and position of the body.

Muscle spindles are specialized structures embedded in each muscle that are proprioceptive (in this case, sensitive to changes in length), i.e., they respond to a sudden stretch, reflexively causing contraction (stretch reflex). Golgi tendon organs are located near the musculo-tendinous junction and are sensitive to changes in muscle tension. They inhibit the muscle's potential to develop excessive tension that may cause injury.

Resistance Training Strength Gains

Early gains in strength appear to be more influenced by neural factors, but later long-term gains are almost solely the result of hypertrophy.[30] Neural factors may include:

- recruitment of additional motor units (increasing a muscle's ability to generate force)
- decreased activity from inhibitory Golgi tendon organs
- improved coordination
- improved motor learning

Chronic muscle hypertrophy (increase in fiber size) appears to be related to:

- increased myofibrils
- increased actin and myosin filaments
- increased connective tissue
- increased capillary density
- increased muscle protein synthesis
- high levels of testosterone
- intense resistance training

Whether or not strength gains result from muscle hyperplasia (increase in the number of muscle fibers) remains controversial. Hyperplasia has been shown in animal studies, but human studies have been inconclusive.

In the early stages of resistance training, strength gains are usually more dramatic because of the large genetic potential to be realized. After this period of rapid initial strength gain, improvement continues, but at an increasingly slower rate as an individual gets closer to realizing his/her genetic potential.

Muscle Soreness

Acute muscle soreness occurs during and immediately after exercise and is due to the accumulation of lactate, decreased oxygen, and tissue swelling within the muscle. Delayed onset muscle soreness (DOMS) occurs 24 to 48 hours post-exercise. Theories that explain DOMS include: damage (ruptures and structural changes) to the muscle fibers themselves; inflammation with accompanying increased white blood cell count; and the stimulation of nerve endings as a result of tissue repair activity. DOMS appears to be even more likely after eccentric exercise, where large forces are distributed over relatively small cross-sectional areas of muscle. Training methods that focus on eccentric (negative) muscle actions should be avoided in the initial stages of training, especially with inactive populations. Delayed onset muscle soreness may be perceived as unpleasant and contribute to non-compliance.

Strength Training Guidelines

Muscular strength is defined as the maximum force a muscle or muscle group can generate at one time.

Muscular endurance is the capacity to sustain repeated muscle actions, as in push-ups or sit-ups, or to sustain fixed, static muscle actions for an extended period of time.

Muscle power is the explosive aspect of strength, and is the product of strength and speed of movement. Power = (force x distance)/time. Power is especially important for improved athletic performance.

Muscular fitness is developed by using the overload principle: increasing the intensity (resistance), frequency or duration of the training above the levels normally experienced. Optimal strength gains occur by using weights that promote maximal or near-maximal muscle tension with few repetitions. Optimal endurance gains develop by using lighter weights with a large number of repetitions. For safe and effective improvement in both muscle strength and endurance, 8 to 12 repetitions at 70–80% of maximum resistance is recommended.

The American College of Sports Medicine recommends the following guidelines for resistance training for the average healthy adult:

Strength and Endurance Continuum

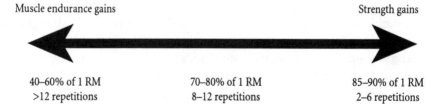

Muscle endurance gains   Strength gains

40–60% of 1 RM   70–80% of 1 RM   85–90% of 1 RM
>12 repetitions   8–12 repetitions   2–6 repetitions

- Perform a minimum of one set. Multiple-set regimens may provide greater benefits if time allows.

- Most people should complete 8–12 repetitions for each exercise to the point of near fatigue. 10–15 repetitions are recommended for frail or elderly people, and for those mostly interested in muscular endurance.

- Perform 8-10 exercises that condition the major muscle groups.
- Perform these exercises a minimum of two to three days per week.

Major muscle groups—Listed here in opposing pairs, they include the: 1) quadriceps and hamstrings, 2) pectoralis major and posterior deltoid, mid-trapezius and rhomboids, 3) deltoids and latissimus dorsi, 4) biceps and triceps, and 5) abdominals and erector spinae. Muscle imbalance occurs and risk of injury increases if only a few muscle groups are trained.

Frequency—Although somewhat greater strength gains can be made by training three days per week, studies show that two days per week also elicits a significant improvement in strength and may be more practical for the general population. Since resistance training can produce cellular microtrauma that can lead to muscle soreness and temporary reductions in strength, adequate rest and recovery time is necessary. Waiting 48 hours between resistance training sessions is a good guideline (longer recovery time may be necessary after very intense workouts). For those who prefer to train every day, avoid working the same muscle groups on consecutive days.

Sets—Studies show that performing a single set to fatigue can result in up to a 25% improvement in strength.[32,33] This is similar to the improvement that occurs from a multi-set program. Single sets may help with exercise adherence since several exercises can be performed in a short amount of time. Programs lasting more than 60 minutes per session are associated with higher dropout rates. However, clients who enjoy weight training and/or need additional calorie expenditure may prefer a multi-set routine (although aerobic conditioning activities are more efficient at calorie expenditure than weight training, per unit of time).

Repetitions and intensity—Most clients can complete 8–12 controlled repetitions with about 75% of their maximum resistance or 1 RM (exercising to the point of fatigue). The higher the resistance, the lower the number of repetitions that can be completed; the lower the resistance, the greater the number of repetitions that are possible (see the strength and endurance continuum above). Also, training at very high intensities increases the risk of injury and may decrease exercise compliance.

Order of exercises—Training the larger muscle groups first is recommended when working with the general public. For example, if the biceps (smaller muscles) were fatigued first, the ability to fatigue the latissimus dorsi (larger muscles) would be limited since the biceps are needed in most latissimus dorsi exercises. Many advocate performing structural exercises (e.g., squats) before isolated body part exercises (e.g., knee extensions) to enhance safety and effectiveness. Abdominal and erector spinae muscles are needed as stabilizers in many exercises, so it makes sense not to exercise them to the point of fatigue until the end of a workout.

Progression—Progressive resistance exercise (PRE) means that resistance must be gradually, progressively increased (overloaded) as the muscles adapt to a given exercise. The double progressive approach works well with most clients: begin with a resistance they can perform eight times to fatigue and as they improve, gradually increase the number of repetitions up to 12. When they can easily perform 12 repetitions, increase the weight (usually about 5%), and that will reduce the number of repetitions back to about eight.

Speed—Although fast lifting may be appropriate for some competitive athletes, risk of injury is increased and it is more difficult to monitor form. For most clients, slow, controlled movement is recommended. Many prefer two seconds for the concentric (shortening) phase and four seconds for the eccentric (lengthening) phase. High intensity work and rapid movement during the eccentric phase have been linked to muscle soreness.

Breathing—To avoid the Valsalva maneuver and the accompanying rise in blood pressure, regular, continuous breathing is important. "Exhaling on the exertion" (or concentric phase) is a good recommendation for most exercises.

Specificity—Specificity is an important concept in fitness training. It refers to the specific adaptations in the metabolic and neuromuscular systems depending on the type of program or exercises that are performed. In strength training, for example, research shows that results are specific to the range of motion trained.[32] It is recommended that exercises be performed through the full range of motion for maximum benefit.

Also, the effect of exercise training is specific to the area of the body being trained; training the upper body has very little effect on the lower body, and vice versa.

In athletic performance, the muscles must be trained with movements as close as possible to the desired movement or skill for optimal results.

Functional exercise—The concept of functional exercise simply refers to the idea that muscles should be trained and developed in such a way as to make the performance of everyday activities easier, smoother, safer and more efficient. In other words, attention should be given to exercises that enhance everyday movements, and thereby improve a client's ability to "function independently" in the real world. For example, a squat is a closed chain (foot is on the floor and weight-bearing) multi-muscle exercise closely resembling the lower body movement patterns in everyday, real-life activities (i.e., getting up and down out of a chair, into and out of a car, and lifting objects off the floor). Many experts advocate moving from isolation-type exercises (e.g., knee extensions) to functional exercises (e.g., squats) as fitness and body awareness improves. A related concept in functional exercise is training the core for stability, since that is what is required in everyday life.

Equipment

Resistance training equipment falls into three main categories:

■ dynamic constant resistance

■ dynamic variable resistance

■ isokinetic

With dynamic (isotonic) constant resistance equipment the external resistance or weight does not vary through the range of motion. Barbells and dumbbells provide constant resistance; if you lift a 20-pound dumbbell, it remains 20 pounds throughout the exercise.

Dynamic variable resistance equipment attempts to match the external resistance to the exerciser's strength curve. Strength varies throughout the range of motion for each muscle. For example, the biceps brachii can exert maximal strength at approximately 100 of elbow flexion, but is much weaker at 60° and at 180° (the end ranges.) This is due both to the angle of pull of the muscle and to the muscle's length-tension relationship. (Maximal tension can be produced when the sarcomeres are at an optimal length, and all myosin cross-bridges connect with actin filaments.) Because of the differences in strength throughout the range of motion, the heaviest constant weight that can be lifted can be no heavier than the weight that can be lifted at the weakest point of the muscle. Variable resistance equipment is designed to compensate for this problem. Cams, moving levers, pulleys, air resistance, etc. are used to alter the resistance through the range of motion, ideally providing maximal tension at all joint angles. Nautilus®, Bodymaster®, Icarion®, Camstar®, Cybex® and Keiser® are a few examples of manufacturers who make variable resistance equipment.

Isokinetic resistance equipment maintains constant muscle tension at a constant speed or velocity. This preset speed cannot be suddenly increased; any force applied against the equipment results in an equal reaction force. Theoretically, muscles could contract maximally through the full range of motion. This premise, as well as the fact that the controlled speed enhances safety, makes isokinetic equipment popular with both elite athletes and physical therapists (it is usually found in rehabilitation centers).

Advantages and disadvantages of the three types of resistance training equipment are shown on the following page.

Types of Resistance Training Equipment

	Constant Resistance	Variable Resistance	Isokinetic Resistance
Examples	Barbells, Dumbbells	Nautilus®, Bodymaster®	Cybex® Rehab
Advantages	• simple, easy to use, relatively inexpensive • requires balance resulting in better coordination and greater muscle utilization • provides for greater variability • easy to maintain, take up very little space • exercises resemble real-life movements	• safe, easy to use • good for beginners because less balance is required • productivity in a short amount of time • requires less supervision • ideal for circuit training	• safe, easy to use • excellent for rehabilitation • intense workout in a short amount of time • detailed performance feedback
Disadvantages	• requires strength to maintain balance and coordination • accidents are more likely to happen • spotters are required • complete workouts may take up more time • inability to train through full range of motion in many exercises • poor matching of resistance to strength curve	• lack of development of balance and coordination • constrained movement patterns • machines are expensive • machines take up a lot of space	• lack of development of balance and joint strength • lack of variety • muscles are worked in isolation • machines are very expensive • machines take up a lot of space • lack of accessibility • some lack ability to perform eccentric contractions

Other types of resistance training techniques include isometric training and plyometrics.

Isometric (static) resistance training involves contracting a muscle in a held position (no change in the joint angle), usually against a wall, weight machine, or against another part of the body. Increases in strength and endurance have been shown from isometric training,[31] especially when the contractions are held for at least six seconds with a maximal effort, and several contractions per day are performed. Isometric training is a common modality in rehabilitation, as it helps maintain strength without excessive joint movement. However, there are several disadvantages to isometric exercises, including: strength gains are joint angle specific (if the exercise is performed at 45° strength gains will occur at 45°, but not necessarily at other joint angles); isometric exercise does not increase motor performance ability; can be time consuming and monotonous; and may cause blood pressure elevation. The rise in blood pressure occurs when the held contraction is accompanied by the Valsalva maneuver (breath holding while bearing down on the glottis). This may create a potentially dangerous situation for cardiac patients, hypertensives, and pregnant women. All clients must be reminded to breathe if isometric exercises are performed.

Plyometric training involves using the stretch reflex to increase fiber recruitment.[87] Known also as jump, rebound, or power training, plyometric exercises eccentrically load the muscle, and require muscles to explosively contract on the rebound. This type of training is more appropriate for athletes as it helps develop speed and power. However, it should be avoided for deconditioned clients due to the need for increased levels of coordination and the high potential for injury.

Equipment Inventory

Review equipment in your facility. Identify whether the machines provide constant or variable resistance, what exercises can be performed on which machines, types of free weights, etc. and record this information on an Equipment Inventory Form (see Appendix B). Typical weight room equipment might include:

Constant Resistance

Bench press bench (wide uprights for Olympic bar)
Incline bench (adjustable)
Decline bench
Preacher curl
Olympic bar with plates
Standard bar with plates
Collars for bars
EZ curl bar
Dumbbells
Cable set ups with high and/or low pulleys
Flat benches
Slant board
Roman chair
Set up for pull-ups and dips
Smith machine
Squat rack
Lunge box

Leg press
Calf machines (standing, seated, donkey)
Gravitron

Variable Resistance

Chest press machine
Pec Dec machine
Scapular adduction machine
Lateral raise machine
Military press machine
Lat pull-down machine
Lat pull-over machine
Biceps curl machine
Triceps extension machine
Abdominal curl machine (*note whether machine targets abdominals or hip flexors*)
Seated rotary torso machine
Back extension machine
Leg press machine
Knee extension machine
Knee curl machine
Standing multi-hip machine
Seated abduction/adduction machine

Exercises for Major Muscle Groups

1. **Quads, hamstrings and buttocks**
   squats (ballet style, weight room style, front squat, back squat, Smith squat), lunges (stationary, front lunge, side lunge, step back lunge, crane lunge), leg press, box step-ups

2. **Quadriceps**
   knee extension machine, supine knee extensions

3. **Hamstrings and buttocks**
   knee curl machine, butt blaster machine, all fours position leg lifts and knee curls, prone position leg lifts and knee curls, supine buttocks squeezes, dead lift, good morning exercise

4. **Calves**
   standing heel raise, seated heel raise, donkey heel raise, calf machine

5. **Anterior tibialis**
   toe lifts (dorsiflexion) with or without foot weight

6. **Inner and outer thighs**
   seated abductor/adductor machine, side-lying leg lifts (knee bent or straight), standing multi-hip machine, low pulley

7. **Deltoids**
   lateral raises, overhead press, upright rows, front raises (anterior), reverse flys and horizontal rows (posterior)

8. **Latissimus dorsi**
   bent over rows, seated rows in sagittal plane, lat pull-down machine, chin-ups, lat pull-over machine

9. **Pectoralis major**
   push-ups, bench press (flat, incline, decline), chest press machine, dumbbell flys (flat, incline, decline), pec dec, cable crossovers

10. **Trapezius and rhomboids**
    prone dorsal lifts, reverse flys on flat or incline bench, reverse flys standing w/cable cross-over or tubing, horizontal seated row, scapular adduction machine

11. **Biceps**
    dumbbell curls (standing, seated, alternating, supine, incline bench, etc.), preacher curls, concentration curls, hammer curls, biceps machine

12. **Triceps**
    bent over elbow extensions, French press, standing press downs (lat machine or high pulley), push-ups, triceps machine, dips, supine elbow extensions

13. **Rotator cuff**
    standing or seated internal and external rotation with band or tube, side-lying or prone external rotation, supine internal rotation, rotary shoulder machine

14. **Forearms**
    supinated wrist curls, pronated wrist curls, curls with wrist roller, hand grips and squeezes, forearm machine

15. **Abdominals**
    supine crunches and crunch twists (incline, flat or decline), crunches with legs up (in air, on wall or bench), supine posterior pelvic tilts (feet on floor or elevated), combo curls, abdominal machine (make sure spinal flexion, not hip flexion, is performed)

16. Erector spinae

seated low back machine, prone hyperextension (one arm, both arms, opposite arm and leg), all fours hyperextension ↶ isometric hold (opposite arm and leg lifted), Roman chair back extensions, dead lifts

Flexibility

Flexibility is the ability of the tissues surrounding a joint to yield to stretching and then to relax and elongate. It is also defined as the range of motion possible around a joint. Flexibility is joint specific and joint-action specific. It is perhaps the most ignored and misused component of fitness.

Benefits of Flexibility Include:

- decreased risk of injury
- decreased stress
- decreased chronic muscle tension
- improved postural awareness
- increased mind/body connection
- relief of muscle soreness[34]
- decreased low back pain
- increased motor performance
- increased self-discipline
- improved ability to perform activities of daily living (increased functional ability)

Factors influencing flexibility

Muscular relaxation is passive; muscles relax when they no longer receive nerve impulses to contract. They "let go." However, muscle fibers cannot elongate by themselves. They need to be placed in an elongated position by the contraction of the antagonistic muscles on the other side of the joint, or by another part of the body, another person, etc. For optimal stretching, have the muscle elongate in the opposite direction from its concentric contraction, and place the body in a position in which the muscle is supported so that it can relax. For example, the hamstrings are responsible for hip extension and knee flexion (the concentric phase of contraction), and therefore, to elongate them, the joints need to be placed in hip flexion and knee extension. Then, the body must be placed in a non-weight bearing position in which the hamstrings can "let go" and relax, such as a seated hamstring stretch in which the upper body is supported by the hands on the floor.

The joint capsule, ligaments, tendons, fascia and skin can all contribute significantly to lack of range of motion around a joint. Flexibility can also be restricted by the shape and contour of the bony joint surfaces (these are usually genetically determined), and by changes within the joint such as bony spurs or arthritis. Women tend to be more flexible than men, and younger people tend to be more flexible than older people. Increasing age, especially coupled with inactivity, typically results in more rigid connective tissue and an adaptive shortening of the muscle fibers. Muscle and tendon temperature affect flexibility; elevations in core temperature of as little as one degree can increase muscle elasticity and decrease connective tissue resistance.

Types of Stretching

Ballistic stretching

Ballistic stretching is characterized by bouncing, pulsing, rapid, or uncontrolled type movements. Although ballistic stretching may be appropriate for certain athletic warm-ups as preparation for specific performance movements, the risk of injury outweighs the benefit for most exercisers. Ballistic stretching has the potential of invoking the stretch (myotatic) reflex. Muscle spindles (sensitive to sudden changes in muscle length) can trigger a reflex contraction after being rapidly, suddenly stretched. This creates more tension in the muscle and may lead to injury.

Static stretching

Static stretching is characterized by low intensity, long duration muscle elongation, ideally in a relaxed and supported position. Static stretching has been shown to help provide relief from delayed onset muscle soreness and to have a much lower risk of injury. Static stretching is the most commonly recommended method of stretching.

Active and passive stretching

Some professionals categorize stretching according to what muscles are contracting and whether or not another person is assisting the stretch. Active stretching can be either static or ballistic, and is a type of stretching one performs alone, using the concentric contraction of the opposing muscles. For example, one way to stretch the pectoral muscles is to actively contract the scapular adductors (mid-trapezius and rhomboids), and the posterior deltoids. In passive stretching, the stretch is initiated by another person or outside force (i.e., traction), and the person being stretched is passive. This type of stretching carries a greater risk of injury because the person applying the force cannot feel the sensations of the person being stretched, and therefore, is generally not recommended for personal fitness trainers to perform. (If you have special training in physical therapy, massage therapy, or chiropractic, passively stretching your clients may be more appropriate.)

Proprioceptive neuromuscular facilitation (PNF)

PNF is defined as a method "promoting or hastening the neuromuscular responses through stimulation of the proprioceptors."[35] PNF utilizes several complex principles, including reciprocal inhibition (when the agonist contracts, the antagonist relaxes), as well as the reflex responses of the proprioceptors, especially the Golgi tendon organs (GTOs). By isometrically contracting the muscle that is to be stretched, the GTOs (which are sensitive to changes in tension) allow the muscle to relax and move through an increased range of motion. Proponents of PNF cite research showing that PNF is more effective than other types of stretching, may help "reset" the stretch reflex level, and creates more strength, balance and stability around a joint. Disadvantages of PNF include the possibility of the Valsalva maneuver (during the isometric contraction), the increased risk of injury when a partner (or trainer) is used, and the increased risk of injury even when performed individually due to the increased tension occurring in the muscles.

PNF was originally used to describe a method of therapy using spiral-diagonal patterns of movement. PNF stretching involves a variety of techniques. Some of the most common methods include:

Hold-relax (HR)—The muscle to be stretched is placed in its lengthened position and isometrically contracts while the partner attempts to move the limb into a deeper stretch. The stretcher then relaxes, and the limb is moved passively into the new range by the partner or by the stretcher.

Contract-relax (CR)—This stretching technique is similar to hold-relax. The difference is that the partner provides an immovable resistance while the stretcher isometrically contracts the muscle to be stretched and attempts to move the limb into the shortened range of the target muscle. The stretcher then relaxes, and the limb is moved passively into the new range by the stretcher.[36]

Contract-relax, antagonist-contract (CRAC)—Begin with the contract-relax method described above, and then, the stretcher, following the isometric contraction of the muscle being stretched, actively contracts the opposing muscle, moving the limb into the new range of motion.

Flexibility Training Guidelines

Always warm up prior to stretching.

Frequency—Three to five stretching sessions per week are adequate for most clients to maintain flexibility. For improvement, some clients will need to stretch more frequently; daily or even twice daily if the goal is to become proficient in a discipline such as hatha yoga. Also, some experts recommend repeating stretches within a stretching session (e.g., performing a hamstring stretch three times).

Intensity—For static and PNF stretching, the intensity should be just below the pain threshold. A sensation of stretch should be felt, without experiencing pain.

Duration—For flexibility gains, a long duration stretch is best. Many sources recommend 10 to 30 seconds for practical reasons, but studies show that the longer a stretch is held, the greater the increases in flexibility. In practices such as hatha yoga, stretches may be held for several minutes.

Breathing—Slow, deep diaphragmatic breathing with the emphasis on the exhale is very relaxing and helps facilitate the mind/body connection. Instead of having clients count seconds (e.g., 10-30), try having them count three to five slow, deep breaths, visualizing the muscles letting go on each exhale, and allowing the stretch to go deeper with each breath.

Muscles to be stretched—Just as with resistance training, 8 to 10 major muscles should be stretched after a workout, especially areas that are commonly tight, such as hamstrings, erector spinae, hip flexors, calves, pectoralis major and anterior deltoids.

Exercises Not Recommended for the General Public According to AFAA and/or Other Major Organizations

- ballistic stretches
- deep squats (knee bends)
- hurdler's stretch
- yoga plow
- unsupported forward flexion of the lumbar spine
- unsupported forward flexion with rotation (of the lumbar spine) unsupported lateral flexion of the lumbar spine
- hyperextension of the cervical spine
- percussive (ballistic) lumbar hyperextension
- side-lying "L" position for hip abduction
- full straight leg sit-ups
- V sits
- double leg raises
- full cobra

During aerobic dance:

- high-impact jumping without bringing the heels down
- hopping more than eight times in a row on one leg

- improper footwear
- ankle weights
- excessive numbers of musculoskeletal high stress moves in a row
- forced high kicks
- improper intensity for level of participant

Other Poor Technique and Alignment Problems

- hyperextended joints
- excessive use of momentum
- overshooting of toes (hyperflexed knee in weight-bearing position)
- knee torque (twisting of tibia relative to femur)
- excessive lordosis, excessive kyphosis, forward head
- excessive ankle pronation or supination

Exercise Analysis: Use the Following AFAA Five Questions™

1. What muscle(s) are you trying to stretch, limber or strengthen? (What is the purpose of the exercise or movement?)

2. Are you doing that? (Are you actually stretching, limbering or strengthening the target muscle(s)? Is the exercise effective? Look at the moving joints to analyze the prime movers.)

   For strength exercises:
   – is the muscle you are trying to train the prime mover?
   – is there resistance applied?
   – is there full range of motion?
   – is the muscle isolated?

   For stretching exercises:
   – is the muscle elongated across the joints?
   – is the muscle relaxed?
   – is the limb supported?

3. Is the back protected, and are there any other stress points? (Is the exercise safe?)

4. Can you isolate the muscle(s) and stay in alignment?

5. For whom is the exercise appropriate or inappropriate? Can this exercise or discipline be modified to accommodate the skill and experience level of the individual or class?

In addition, the following Exercise Grid may help you "break down" an exercise.

Exercise Grid				
Name of exercise	What joints are moving?	What is the joint action?	What plane?	What muscle(s) are prime movers for that joint action?
Example: Bench Press	shoulders	shoulder horizontal	horizontal	anterior deltoid pectoralis major
	elbows	elbow extension		triceps

IN SUMMARY

This chapter covered benefits of strength and endurance training, muscle structure, strength training guidelines, advantages and disadvantages of different types of resistance training equipment and exercises for major muscle groups. In addition, flexibility benefits, types of stretching, and flexibility training guidelines were given. Higher risk exercises and technique problems were listed in addition to guides for helping to determine the safety and effectiveness of an exercise.

Chapter 7

Nutrition and Weight Management

Since poor nutrition and obesity are implicated in many chronic diseases, personal fitness trainers have a responsibility to provide educational information about the fundamentals of a healthy diet whenever it is appropriate. Scientists estimate that 40% of all cancer incidence in men, and 60% in women, is related to diet. In addition, high cholesterol, high blood pressure, adult-onset diabetes, and obesity are all related to poor quality nutrition. While clients with special dietary needs and problems must be referred to a registered dietitian (trainers must beware of "prescribing a diet"), information that is in the public domain, such as the Food Guide Pyramid and the recommendations from the American Heart Association, can and should be taught.

The USDA Food Guide Pyramid (1992) prioritizes food groups to help ensure that people obtain their RDAs (Recommended Dietary Allowances). Even though nutrient and calorie needs vary from person to person, depending on age, gender, size and physical activity level, most adults should try to eat at least the lower number of servings from each food group. Many athletes (and most men) can have the middle to upper number of servings.

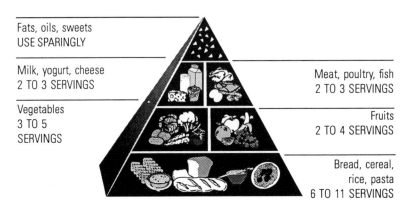

Fats, oils, sweets
USE SPARINGLY

Milk, yogurt, cheese
2 TO 3 SERVINGS

Vegetables
3 TO 5
SERVINGS

Meat, poultry, fish
2 TO 3 SERVINGS

Fruits
2 TO 4 SERVINGS

Bread, cereal,
rice, pasta
6 TO 11 SERVINGS

Food Guide Pyramid

Food Group	Suggested Daily Servings	What Counts as a Serving?
Breads, cereals and other grain products	6–11 servings; include several servings of whole-grain products daily	1 slice of bread; hamburger bun or English muffin; a small roll or muffin; 3-4 small, or 2 large, crackers; 1/2 cup cooked cereal, rice or pasta; 1 oz. cold cereal
Fruits (citrus, melons, berries, other fruits)	2–4 servings	A whole fruit such as a medium apple, banana or orange; a grapefruit half; a melon wedge; 3/4 cup of juice; 1/2 cup of of berries; 1/4 cup of dried fruit
Vegetables (dark green leafy, deep yellow, dry beans and peas, starchy vegetables)	3–5 servings; include all types regularly; use dark green leafy vegetables and dry beans and peas several times a week	1/2 cup of cooked vegetables; 1/2 cup chopped raw vegetables; 1 cup of leafy raw vegetables, such as lettuce or spinach
Meat, poultry, fish and alternatives (eggs, dry beans and peas, nuts, seeds)	2–3 servings	Amounts should total 5–7 oz. of cooked lean meat, poultry or fish a day. Count 1 egg, 1/2 cup cooked beans, or 2 T. of peanut butter as 1 oz. of meat.
Milk, cheese, and yogurt (low or non-fat types)	2–3 servings	1 cup of milk; 8 oz. of yogurt; 1 1/2 oz. of natural cheese; 2 oz. of processed cheese
Fats, sweets, and alcoholic beverages	Avoid too many fats and sweets. If you drink alcoholic beverages, do so in moderation.	1 oz. of pure alcohol equals: 12-oz. beers, two small glasses or wine, or 1 1/2 fluid oz. of spirits

Have your clients write down everything they eat for three typi͜ days (three-day dietary recall) and then see if they are meeting their minir͞ ͞ daily requirements according to the Food Guide Pyramid.

American Heart Association Guidelines

The AHA recommends that daily caloric intake consist of:

■ 55–60% carbohydrates with no more than 15% from simple carbohydrates

■ 10–12% protein

■ <30% fat with <10% saturated fat

Carbohydrates

Carbohydrates are the body's main source of energy. There are two main types: simple carbohydrates (sugars, including glucose and fructose from fruit and vegetables, lactose from milk, and sucrose from cane or beet sugar) and complex carbohydrates (i.e., carrots, broccoli, corn, potatoes, bread, cereal, pasta, rice and beans), which contain glucose, fiber and many other nutrients. For active exercisers, consuming 60% of daily calories from carbohydrates is important. If you are consuming 2,000 calories per day, then 60% would equal 1,200 calories from carbohydrates. Since there are four calories in one gram of carbohydrates, you would need to consume 300 grams of carbohydrates per day. Read labels and help yourself and your clients have enough daily energy!

Fiber

There are two types of fiber: soluble and insoluble. Soluble fiber is found in fruits, vegetables, seeds, brown rice, barley and oats. It appears to lower blood cholesterol levels and retard the entry of glucose into the bloodstream. Insoluble fiber includes cellulose, and is found mainly in whole grains and on the outside of seeds, fruits, and legumes. Insoluble fiber is key in promoting more efficient elimination and is thought to play a role in colon cancer prevention. The daily recommendation for fiber is 20–30 grams per day.

Protein

Protein is essential for building and repairing muscles, red blood cells, hair and other tissues, and is necessary for synthesizing hormones. Protein is digested into twenty-two amino acids, thirteen of which the body manufactures. Since the human body cannot manufacture the other nine amino acids, they are known as essential. A "complete" protein (such as animal or fish based foods) supplies these essential amino acids. An "incomplete" protein lacks one or more of the essential amino acids. These incomplete proteins are generally from plants (e.g., fruits, grains and vegetables). By combining grains with legumes (e.g., dried beans or tofu with rice or bread), the nine essential amino acids can still be obtained without necessarily eating animal products. The RDA for protein for adults is 0.8–1.0 grams of protein for each kilogram (2.2 pounds) of body weight. This correlates fairly well with the AHA guideline of 10–12% of daily calories from protein. There are four calories in one gram of protein.

To Calculate Protein Needs:

1. Calculate your weight in kilograms: body weight in pounds x .45 = body weight in kilograms
2. Multiply weight in kilograms by either 0.8 or 1.0 (or both numbers for a range). The result is the grams of protein you should consume per day.

Another recommendation for consuming adequate, but not excess, protein in your diet is to include two cups of low-fat or skim milk or yogurt plus five to seven ounces of protein rich foods per day.

Government surveys show that Americans typically consume about 100 grams of protein a day—nearly twice as much as the RDA[37], and that most of this protein comes from meat sources. Meat is a primary source of saturated fats (which are the major culprit in elevated cholesterol levels); diets high in meat but not dairy products increase the loss of calcium in the body. High protein diets also stress the kidneys, may cause diarrhea, and worsen dehydration. Athletes today are still (literally) buying into the myth that they require large amounts of protein to increase muscle mass, and spend large sums of money on powdered protein supplements or amino acid tablets. Most authorities agree that even professional athletes don't need extra protein if their caloric intake is adequate. Studies of athletes have not found that protein supplements improve strength, power or endurance. Also, excess protein in the body is usually turned into fat, not muscle.

Fat

Fat adds flavor to food, and is an important component of a healthy diet. Fat is necessary for energy production, transporting fat soluble vitamins, protection of internal organs, insulation, healthy skin and hair, and for supplying the "essential" fat, linoleic acid. Unfortunately, Americans eat almost twice as much fat as the human body is designed to handle; up to 36% to 41% of total daily calories often comes from fat.[38] A high fat diet has been linked in numerous studies to increased risk of heart disease, cancer, diabetes, and other problems. It is also a major contributor to obesity and all its associated ills. Less than 30% (some authorities say less than 25%) of total daily calories should come from fat. Fat is more than twice as fattening as proteins or carbohydrates, with nine calories in one gram of fat.

Types of fat

Triglycerides are the main type of fat found in the diet and in adipose tissue. Desirable levels are under 200 mg/dl.

Saturated fats come primarily from animal sources and include: butter, whole milk dairy products, and meats. Hamburger is the largest contributor to saturated fat intake in the American diet, with cheese ranking second. Coconut and palm oils are also highly saturated. Vegetable oil margarines become partially saturated when they are hydrogenated, making them solid at room temperature (which is why liquid oils and soft tub margarines are preferable to stick margarines). Saturated fat raises cholesterol levels more than anything else in the diet.[39] Less than 10% of daily calories should come from saturated fat sources.

Unsaturated fats can be either monounsaturated or polyunsaturated.

- **Monounsaturated fats** have been shown to reduce LDL cholesterol without affecting the beneficial HDLs, and are therefore the preferred form of fat in the diet. Good sources include olive oil, canola oil, peanut oil and avocado oil.

- **Polyunsaturated fats** are divided into the omega-6 vegetable oils and the omega-3 fish oils. The vegetable oils include sunflower, corn and sesame. The omega-3 oils come primarily from fish, especially mackerel, halibut, salmon, albacore tuna and whitefish. Omega-3 oils have been shown to suppress atherosclerosis in animal studies[40], and to decrease blood pressure, cholesterol, triglycerides and blood clotting.

Cholesterol is actually not a fat at all; it is an "alcohol wax" that at times behaves like a fat. It is a natural compound found in all animal tissues. It is essential for life, so much so that the human body manufactures all it needs without any help from dietary cholesterol. Cholesterol is also important as a structural component of cell membranes and blood lipids, and in the production of hormones and bile (aids in the digestion of fat). Eating cholesterol-rich foods is not the primary cause of high cholesterol; a high fat diet, especially one high in saturated fats, is the major cause. Nevertheless the AHA recommends that no more than 300 milligrams of cholesterol be eaten per day.

All fats and oils have nine calories per gram of fat, and contain about 14 grams of fat which equals approximately 120 calories per tablespoon. "Healthful oils" have the highest proportions of unsaturated fat to saturated fat. The real key, however, is to cut down on all fats, as high total levels of dietary fat leave little room for other healthful foods (such as carbohydrates), and are linked with obesity and other negative health outcomes.

To figure the maximum amount of fat your client should be eating, estimate how many calories he/she consumes each day and multiply by 30%. Divide that number by nine to figure grams of fat per day.

Total caloric intake	Total calories from fat	Grams of fat
1,200	360	40
1,500	450	50
1,800	540	60
2,000	600	66
2,500	750	83

Help clients cut back on fat. Teach them to:

1. Read labels. Determine both the amount and type of fats in foods. To determine the number of calories that come from fat, multiply the grams of fat in a serving by nine. Divide this number by the total calories in the serving to get the percentage of calories coming from fat.

2. Substitute fish or chicken (skinless) for some red meat.

3. Eat more meatless meals. Use vegetables, grains and legumes as the main dish.

4. Select lean meats and eat smaller portions (three to five ounces). Trim off all visible fat.

5. Limit intake of fats and oils, especially those high in saturated fat. Choose a margarine that has at least twice as much polyunsaturated fat as saturated.

6. Broil, bake, or boil foods instead of frying.

7. Cut back on fat-laden snack foods, e.g., potato chips, cookies, pastries.

Blood Lipid and Lipoprotein Norms in mg/dl				
	Desirable	**Borderline**	**High Risk**	**Very High**
Total Cholesterol	<200	200–239	>240	
HDL Cholesterol	>35		<35	
LDL Cholesterol	<130	130-159	≥160	
Triglycerides	<200	200–400	400–1,000	>1,000

National Cholesterol Education Program, 1993. JAMA, 269, 23, 3015-23

Label Reading

The new food labels mandated by the Food and Drug Administration for processed foods were on most products as of July, 1994. Single ingredient foods, such as fresh fruits, vegetables, meat, poultry, fish and unprocessed grains are not required to have labels. The new labels must contain the following information.

Mandated Food Label Information			
total calories	calories from fat	total fat	saturated fat
cholesterol	dietary fiber	sodium	total carbohydrates
sugars	protein	vitamin A	vitamin C
calcium	iron		

Sample of new food labeling format:

Nutrition Facts

Serving size 6 cookies (28g)
Servings per container about 11

Amount per Serving

Calories 120	Calories from Fat 36

%Daily Value*

Total Fat 4g	**6%**
Saturated Fat 0.5g	**4%**
Polyunsaturated Fat 0g	
Monounsaturated Fat 1g	
Cholesterol 5mg	**2%**
Sodium 105mg	**4%**
Total Carbohydrate 20g	**7%**
Dietary Fiber less than 1g	**2%**
Sugars 7g	
Protein 2g	

Vitamin A 0%

Vitamin C 0% • Calcium 0% • Iron 8%

*Percent Daily Values are based on a 2,000 calorie diet. Your daily values may be higher or lower depending on your calorie needs:

	Calories	2,000	2,500
Total Fat	less than	66g	83g
Sat Fat	Less than	20g	25g
Cholesterol	Less than	300g	300mg
Sodium	Less than	2,400mg	2,400mg
Total Carbohydrate		300g	375g
Dietary Fiber		25g	30g

Calories Per Gram: Fat 9 • Carbohydrate 4 • Protein 4

When reading labels:

1. Look carefully at the serving size. If your normal serving size is more or less than the serving that is listed, you'll need to adjust when considering the amount of fat (or carbohydrates, or proteins) in the product.

2. Look at the calories from fat. Figure the percent of calories coming from fat by dividing the total calories into the calories from fat (in the example above: 36 ÷ 120 = 30%).

3. Look at the grams of fat in the food and consider how this food fits into your total daily fat gram allotment.

4. The percentage (%) daily value can be confusing for some clients. It measures the amount of the particular nutrient in the food (e.g., fat) against the amount of that nutrient an average person is supposed to have in one day. So, if you consume a 2,000 calorie per day diet, 30% fat is 600 calories from fat or about 65–66 grams of fat (see bottom of label). A serving of six cookies nets four grams of fat which is 6% of the 66 total grams of fat you are allowed per day.

5. On the bottom of each label is a little nutrition lesson. Teach your clients what these numbers mean. For people consuming 2,000 or 2,500 calories per day, total fat, saturated fat, cholesterol, sodium, total carbohydrate, and dietary fiber recommendations are right there. In addition, calorie values per gram of fat, carbohydrates, and protein are on the labels for easy reference.

Vitamins and Minerals

Vitamins are either fat soluble (A,D,E,K) or water soluble (C, B complex) and are essential to catalyze chemical reactions in the body. Minerals are classed as either major (e.g., calcium, phosphorus) or minor (zinc, copper) and are needed to regulate body processes. Vitamins and minerals have no caloric value and cannot provide energy.

Nutrient Density

Nutrient density is the concept of eating foods that are very nutritious relative to the number of calories. Specifically, a high nutrient-dense food provides at least 5% of the RDA of one or more nutrients at a modest caloric cost (e.g., broccoli). At the other end of the spectrum, a food low in nutrient density provides a small amount of nutrition relative to the calories (e.g., potato chips). Usually, foods high in fat, sugar or alcohol are low in nutrient density. During certain phases of life and for some populations, eating nutrient-dense foods is especially important. Seniors, children, and people on weight-reduction type diets, as well as pregnant or breast-feeding women, can't afford to waste many of their calories on low nutrient-dense (junk) foods. Examples of high nutrient-dense foods include: spinach, greens, bell peppers, cantaloupe, papaya, brown rice, wheat bran, whole wheat bread, nonfat plain yogurt, skim milk, water-packed tuna and black beans.

Pre- and Post-Exercise Eating

Eating appropriately prior to exercise helps boost carbohydrate energy and minimizes an insulin surge. (High insulin levels in the blood can contribute to low blood sugar and potential hypoglycemia when combined with exercise.) Foods low on the glycemic index, such as apples, oranges and raw carrots make good pre-exercise snacks. The glycemic index is a ranking that measures how much a given carbohydrate (50 grams worth) elevates blood sugar above normal. Several factors are involved in assigning glycemic index values to carbohydrates, including: the food's rate of digestion, fiber content, type of fiber, cooking, ripeness and presence of protein or fat, etc.[41] Foods low on the index provide a prolonged, sustained entry of glucose into the bloodstream.

Conversely, foods high on the glycemic index scale are released more quickly into the blood and are better for recovery and refueling after exercise. It is recommended that you eat at least 50 grams (200 calories) of a high- or moderate-glycemic carbohydrate as soon after exercise as possible.[42] Two hours later, eat another 50 grams or so of a high-glycemic carbohydrate. Bagels, pasta, raisins and baked potatoes are good recovery foods (be sure to limit or omit fats, e.g., butter or cream cheese) on these carbohydrates as fat slows down the release of sugar into the bloodstream. These guidelines are particularly important for endurance athletes and those exercising twice a day.[43] In addition, foods high in electrolytes (minerals such as potassium, calcium and sodium) are important for recovery after prolonged exercise (two or more hours). Good choices include potatoes, low-fat yogurt, bananas and orange juice.

Carbohydrate loading is a pre-event practice used by endurance athletes to maximally load their muscles with stored glycogen. When preparing for marathons or other events lasting more than 90 minutes, it is recommended that: 1) athletes cut back on exercise and rest their muscles prior to competition, and 2) they eat a high-carbohydrate diet (60–70%) for three days prior to the event in order to "supersaturate" the muscles with glycogen.[44]

Hydration

Adequate hydration is important for everyone, but it is especially critical for regular exercisers to replace body fluids, as dehydration is more likely during and after prolonged exercise and can have serious consequences. At the least, dehydration may cause decreased performance, headaches and constant fatigue. Fluid in the body has at least three important functions.

- Fluid in blood transports glucose to working muscles and carries away metabolic by-products.
- Fluid in urine eliminates metabolic waste products.
- Fluid in sweat dissipates heat through the skin.

Recommendations include the following. Check the color and quantity of your urine (it should be clear and copious). Weigh yourself before and after exercise. For every pound of weight lost, drink two cups of fluid. It is hard to over-hydrate before and during exercise: drink one or two cups of water 5 to 15 minutes before your workout, and a minimum of three ounces every 20 minutes of exercise. During hot and humid conditions and during prolonged and/or intense exercise, even more water is required—drink up to 8 to 10 ounces every 20 minutes. After exercise, continue to drink when thirsty, plus more. For exercise bouts lasting longer than 90 minutes, diluted juice and/or a sports drink will add beneficial electrolytes and help maintain blood sugar balance. After prolonged exercise, juice is preferable because of its higher levels of carbohydrates and electrolytes.[44]

Supplements

Between 35% and 40% of American adults take vitamin and mineral supplements (the incidence is even higher among the athletic population).[45] Many believe they provide nutritional "insurance"—that even if breakfast is skipped and a fast food lunch is eaten, supplements constitute a nutritional shortcut. Vitamins and minerals, however, work with other nutrients in food, and cannot overcome a poor diet. No supplement will replace what a high-carbohydrate, moderate-protein, low-fat diet can do for your body. Very few people really need supplements. Those who do should seek the advice of a registered dietitian and include: pregnant women, seniors, those who take aspirin frequently, heavy drinkers, smokers, the chronically ill, vegetarians, those with food allergies, and those on restricted calorie diets. Megadosing (any dose greater than 10 times the RDA), is not only wasteful, but potentially dangerous. Personal fitness trainers should beware of recommending supplementation of any kind to their clients, for legal as well as health reasons. Many people assume that vitamin and mineral products and other ergogenic aids (substances used to enhance performance) do what they are advertised to do. In fact, many distributors of supplements use questionable marketing techniques including:

- using invalid or inappropriate research and taking advantage of consumers' ignorance about research methodology and applications

- suggesting that there is a need for a particular product when in fact there is no need

- using endorsement by professional organizations or groups without their full or informed consent

- using testimonials instead of peer-reviewed, controlled studies

- using a patent number as if it were a government endorsement (which it is not)
- misleading consumers by making advertisements appear to be news stories
- promoting the myth that if a little is good, a lot is even better

When evaluating claims, be sure they have been substantiated in a reputable, peer-reviewed scientific journal. Determine if the claim has been studied by other credible researchers and whether or not the same results were achieved. Look for research studies carried out by scientists using objective methods, without financial connections to the end result. (Who paid for the study?) If it was a long-term study, a control group should have been utilized. Finally, if the claim sounds too good to be true, it probably is!

Antioxidants

There is mounting evidence suggesting that high dosages of the antioxidant vitamins (C,E and beta-carotene) are linked to the prevention of heart disease, cataracts and various cancers, and may have special benefits for active people.[45,46] They are called antioxidants because they appear to neutralize a class of atomic particles known as "free radicals" (unstable oxygen molecules created during normal cellular metabolism that can cause structural damage to the cells themselves). Most people can get enough vitamin C and beta-carotene from food if they eat plenty of citrus fruits and orange, red, yellow and dark green fruits and vegetables. Those with low fat intakes (below 25%) may have trouble getting enough vitamin E. Some sources recommend a supplement with no more than five to six milligrams of beta-carotene and about 250 milligrams each of vitamins C and E.[47] Remember that the fat-soluble vitamins A, D, E and K are toxic when taken in high doses. Watch for additional research in this area.

Eating Disorders

How do you know when food obsessions cross over into eating disorders? According to the *Diagnostic and Statistical Manual of Mental Disorders*, criteria for anorexia nervosa include:

- intense fear of becoming obese, which does not diminish as weight loss progresses
- disturbance of body image, i.e. claiming to "feel fat" even when emaciated
- weight loss of at least 15% of original body weight
- refusal to maintain body weight over a minimal normal weight for age and height
- no known physical illness that would account for the weight loss

Other symptoms of anorexia include: hyperactivity, compulsive exercising, loss of hair, amenorrhea (loss of menstrual periods), growth of fine body hair, extreme sensitivity to cold temperatures, feeling of being nervous at mealtime, denial, wearing clothing several sizes too large (due to the anorexic's perception that she is too large to fit into smaller sizes).

Criteria for bulimia nervosa include:

- recurrent episodes of binge eating
- consumption of high-calorie, easily ingested food during a binge
- inconspicuous eating during a binge
- binge eating episodes terminating with abdominal pain, sleep or self-induced vomiting
- repeated attempts to lose weight with severely restrictive diets, self-induced vomiting, or use of diuretics
- weight fluctuations of greater than 10 pounds due to alternating binges and fasts
- depressed mood and self-deprecating thoughts following eating binges

Other symptoms of bulimia include: frequent vomiting, damage to throat, bursting blood vessels in eyes, loss of tooth enamel, secretive behavior, excessive concern with physical appearance, and difficulty swallowing and retaining food.

Research shows that these disorders are on the rise, especially among young, college age women athletes. In one study, 3% of 690 athletes in Midwestern colleges met the diagnostic criteria for anorexia, and 21.5% met the criteria for bulimia.[48] Eating disorders and amenorrhea are part of the "Female Athlete Triad," along with osteoporosis. These three related problems can have serious, long-term repercussions for women. According to the American College of Sports Medicine, women with one component of the Triad should be screened for the other components.

Internal and external pressures placed on girls and women to achieve or maintain an unrealistic body weight (in this case, an extremely low body weight) underlies the development of these disorders.[96] Fitness professionals should emphasize health and total well-being, not weight.

Helping clients with eating disorders may be difficult. According to the American Dietetic Association, nutrition education and intervention should be integrated into a team approach for individuals with anorexia, bulimia and binge eating (or compulsive overeating) disorder. If you suspect that a friend or client has a disorder, be supportive and nonjudgemental. Try to build a bond of trust, which may help the person to be more receptive to your suggestions for help. Have available a referral to a health professional qualified to deal with eating disorders.

Note: No such condition should be "treated" by a personal fitness trainer. Instead your client should be referred to an appropriately qualified and licensed health care provider.

Weight Management

Obesity is defined as a level of excess body fat that increases the risk of disease. Specifically, it is having a body weight more than 20% above a desirable level, a body mass index greater than 30, or a percentage of body fat greater than 30% for women and greater than 20% for men. Overweight is defined as a body mass index (BMI = kg/m2) $\geq$27.8 for men and $\geq$27.3 for women. According to recent data from the third National Health and Nutrition Examination Survey, approximately 33% of U.S. adults are overweight.[49] The incidence of overweight tends to be disproportionately high among minority women and women of lower socioeconomic status and/or lower educational level (currently 49% among African-American women and 47% among Mexican-American women[50]).

Obesity constitutes a significant health hazard. It is a contributing risk factor for heart disease, and influences the development of hypertension, diabetes and cholesterol abnormalities. It is a risk factor for certain kinds of cancer. It is associated with gall-stones, gout, respiratory insufficiency, impaired heat tolerance, congestive heart failure, and increased risk from surgery, as well as musculoskeletal problems such as back pain and knee pain.[8] It increases the likelihood of hemorrhoids, hernias and varicose veins. These risks vary depending on genetic predisposition, other risk factors, degree of obesity, fitness level and the location of body fat stores. Fat that is carried in the abdomen and upper body areas poses a greater health risk than extra fat that is stored in the hips and thighs.

Several factors are responsible for obesity, including physical inactivity, poor nutrition, lack of nutrition education, genetics, socioeconomic factors, resting metabolic rate, number of fat cells (adipocytes), psychological factors, and ready availability of poor quality foods. Much research has been devoted to the study of fat cell development, number and size. The body appears to increase its quantity of adipose tissue in two ways: first, by increasing the size (hypertrophy) of existing fat cells (filling them with more fat), and secondly by increasing the number of fat cells (hyperplasia). Obese individuals typically have about twice as many fat cells as those who are not obese, with more fat per cell. This may partly account for the difficulty with weight loss and maintenance—when there is an elevated number of fat cells, they seem to resist shrinkage and do not disappear.

Energy balance is an important concept in weight management. Take in more calories than you expend, and the excess will be stored as adipose tissue. Expend more calories than you consume and there will be a negative energy balance (weight loss). To maintain normal metabolic rate and provide energy for activities of daily living, the American Dietetic Association recommends no less than 1,200 calories per day for women and no less than 1,400 calories per day for men.

Caloric expenditure has three components:

- resting metabolic rate (RMR)
- energy expended with exertion (exercise and activities of daily living)
- the thermic effect of food

The RMR accounts for about 60–75% of daily caloric expenditure and is higher in individuals with a high percentage of lean body mass (fat-free mass). Because of the relationship between RMR and lean body mass, it is important to preserve lean body mass when losing weight (this helps maintain the metabolic rate). Several studies show that severely restricting calories lowers the RMR.[51] Other factors affecting the RMR include: gender, age, height, air temperature and physical activity.

Energy expended with exertion accounts for approximately 20–30% of daily caloric output, and is the easiest component to alter. There are at least three ingredients: activities of daily living (e.g., washing, dressing, eating, driving), bouts of exercise (may be as low-level as gardening or as intense as a 10-mile run), and recovery from exercise. The extra calories expended during recovery are often called EPOC (excess post-oxygen consumption). The amount of extra calories burned during EPOC appears to depend on both the duration and the intensity of the exercise bout, and is usually minor when compared to the amount of calories burned during the exercise itself. Also, heavier people expend more calories with exertion than lighter people.

Many clients have misconceptions about the amount of calories they burn during exercise. They are usually surprised and discouraged to learn that a typical exercise session for the exerciser with average fitness burns only about 300 calories (the more fit you are, the longer, harder, and more often you can exercise).

Typical Calorie Expenditure Values		
Activity (30 minutes)	130 lbs. BW	180 lbs. BW
walking at 3.5 mph, 4% grade	173 cal.	241 cal.
running at 6.0 mph, 0% grade	316 cal.	439 cal.
cycling 10 mph on flat surface	177 cal.	243 cal.
step aerobics, 6" step (124 bpm)	241 cal.	336 cal.
swimming, fast crawl	276 cal.	378 cal.
weight training (depends on length of rest periods between sets)	~150 cal.	~210 cal.

The thermic effect of food refers to the increase in RMR after eating and is roughly equivalent to 10% of the meal's total caloric value. For example, if you ate a 500 calorie meal, about 50 calories would be used for digestion and absorption.

The weight loss industry has traditionally focused on dietary changes and caloric restriction. In the past, few commercial diet centers had exercise facilities or offered exercise programming. This has resulted in temporary success for some; pounds were lost, but in most cases they were regained. Studies show that when exercise accompanies dietary changes, not only is lean body mass preserved, but the weight loss is much more likely to be maintained at six months and 12 months after achieving goal weight than with individuals who dieted but didn't exercise.[52] The presence of an exercise habit appears to predict success in the maintenance of lost weight. A combined program of dietary changes, exercise and behavior modification is recommended for clients who want to lose weight. Several specific guidelines for counseling clients about weight reduction follow.

1. Help clients focus on lifelong weight control strategies. Help them to choose diet modifications and exercise routines that they will adhere to over the long run. The exercise recommendation should be more concerned with adherence than with the specifics of frequency, intensity and duration. With deconditioned and inactive clients it doesn't necessarily matter what exercise they do, as long as they do something. Brainstorm with your client about how to increase his/her physical activity level throughout the day in "non-exercise" endeavors (e.g., using stairs instead of elevators). Remember that high intensity levels have been correlated with decreased adherence, especially for deconditioned exercisers.

2. Teach them that exercise is essential for lifelong weight control and good health. You rarely lose weight and keep it off without daily exercise. Remind clients of the other benefits of exercise, such as

stronger bones, healthier heart, less stress and depression, and higher self-esteem. Have them work towards a balanced exercise program: cardiorespiratory exercise, resistance training, and stretching.

3. Prepare clients for the possibility of a lapse or setback. This is very common when making a major behavior change and should not be interpreted as a failure or as a reason to quit. Teach them to persevere.

4. Be careful when establishing an "ideal weight." This elusive number may be counterproductive and discouraging, and many clients may never actually achieve it. Instead, consider developing a "reasonable weight" based on: the lowest weight the client has been able to maintain in the past (for up to a year), loss and regain history, medical history (at what weight, for instance, did high blood pressure develop). Look at the clients' abilities to control their eating habits, the extent of their social support, and their range of coping skills.

5. Set short-term goals. For example, set a goal of a five-pound weight loss, and when that has been achieved, then set a goal of maintaining the five-pound weight loss for one month. When that has been achieved then set another five-pound weight loss goal, etc.

6. Let clients know that losing even 10 or 15 pounds has positive health benefits. Even a small weight loss can reduce blood pressure, lower LDLs, increase HDLs, and help with blood-sugar regulation. It's preferable to lose 10 pounds and keep it off than to lose 20 pounds and gain it back.

7. Help clients realize that it's hard to eat a healthy diet if they're constantly exposed to poor foods. As much as possible, eliminate high calorie, high fat, nutrient poor foods, as well as junk food stimuli from their environment. Help them shop the perimeter of the grocery store and bring home healthy, satisfying choices. Of course, teach label reading. Several excellent resources exist for clients who don't like to cook and who eat out frequently, as well as for those who enjoy cooking and spend a great deal of time in the kitchen (see Appendix A, under Nutrition). Eating well can be its own immediate reward. Healthy eating does not have to mean deprivation, self-pity, or "eating cardboard." People only believe this because they don't know better. It's entirely possible to eat luxurious, delicious, beautiful meals that satisfy both mind and body, and are at the same time nutritious, wholesome, and low-fat.

8. Have clients keep a food record: what and when they ate, as well as what mood they were in when eating. Do they skip meals? Evaluate their carbohydrate, protein and fat (CPF) balance, as well as the number of servings of important food groups, and total calories and fat grams consumed per day. Teach the concept of nutrient density.

9. With your clients, develop a list of 10 non-food activities for them to do when they're bored, tired, lonely, etc. (e.g., take a bath, meditate, call a friend). Help them find substitute behaviors for eating (e.g., if they always eat snacks while watching TV, substitute exercise, sewing or painting while watching TV).

10. Remember that eating well isn't "all or nothing." It's what you do consistently (some say 80% of the time) that matters.

Gaining Weight

Gaining weight may be a priority for some clients. Nancy Clark, RD, offers these six tips for healthful weight gain[53]:

1. Consistently eat three hearty meals per day; make mealtime a priority.

2. Consistently eat larger than normal portions (e.g., instead of one sandwich at lunch, have two).

3. Eat an extra snack (e.g., a large peanut butter sandwich with a tall glass of milk) before bedtime. Pay attention to mid-morning and mid-afternoon snacks as well.

4. Select higher calorie foods (e.g., cranberry juice instead of orange juice, and split pea soup instead of vegetable soup).

5. Drink lots of juice and milk instead of water.

6. Perform resistance training exercises to build muscle.

Protein supplements and other "mass builders" are expensive and tend to promote misconceptions about muscle building. Increasing muscle mass results from the right kind of exercise and a healthy diet; the energy to exercise and fuel muscle activity is supplied by a diet high in carbohydrates. Extra, less expensive calories can easily come from juices and healthy foods.

IN SUMMARY

In this chapter, fundamental concepts in nutrition were addressed, including: the USDA Food Guide Pyramid, American Heart Association Guidelines for a healthy diet, and carbohydrate, protein and fat specifics. Formulas were given for calculating individual protein needs and percentage of daily dietary fat. Types of fat were covered as well as strategies for cutting back on fat intake. Label reading was discussed step by step. Nutrient density, pre- and post-exercise eating, hydration and nutritional supplements were discussed. In addition, information was provided regarding eating disorders, gaining weight, and helping clients with weight loss/weight management.

Chapter 8

Behavior Modification and Communication Skills

Helping clients change and modify their behavior for wellness maintenance is a continuing challenge for health fitness professionals. Whether the lifestyle change is smoking cessation, alcohol abstinence, weight reduction and better eating habits, less stress, or the adoption of a regular exercise routine, clients who want to change share some common behavior patterns. Behavioral scientists have developed many models to explain these patterns and/or the motives behind change. Two of these models, the Health Behavior Change Model and the Transtheoretical Model, may provide some insight into client behavior.

Health Behavior Change Model

The Health Behavior Change Model is derived from Bandura's Social Learning Theory[54] and divides behavior change into three stages: antecedent, adoption and maintenance.

1. **The antecedent stage** is the initial, pre-activity stage, which outlines all the reasons that a client might have to consider changing. These include:

    –   adequate information about the new behavior (such as booklets, handouts, and clear verbal education)

    –   instructions from a person of authority to change (e.g., a physician instructing a patient to reduce his cholesterol)

    –   observing a role model successfully managing the desired new behavior

- previous experience with the new behavior (Has the client tried exercise before, and if so, was it a positive or negative experience? It is very important to build the client's self-confidence and skill as well as the perception that success can be achieved.)

- increasing the incentives to change (remind the client of all the benefits), and decreasing the barriers or disincentives (e.g., inconvenient time or unpleasant activity)

2. **The adoption stage** is the part of the model where the client actually acts on his/her intention to change, and "tries out" the new behavior (i.e., shows up for the first session with a trainer). Small problems can often overwhelm the client at this stage (such as requiring a physician's clearance or having the right footwear), so clear communication with the trainer about what's expected is critical. It's important to be especially supportive and to help build feelings of self-efficacy (the inner confidence that a person has that he or she will be able to accomplish a task).

3. **At the maintenance stage** the client adheres to the new behavior for a prolonged period of time. Four strategies have been identified for enhancing maintenance[55]:

- monitoring and feedback—clients may be encouraged to keep exercise logs and diaries, but the personal attention of a sincerely interested personal fitness trainer can be a key factor in adherence, especially in the first few months.

- reinforcement or rewards—this can be anything that increases the chance that the behavior will be repeated, e.g., praise during or after the behavior, tangible [external] rewards, such as water bottles, certificates or T-shirts, or intangible reinforcers, such as the client acknowledging that he/she feels better inside (internal reward).

- relapse prevention—preparing the client for the possibility of a lapse or slip is essential to avoid a collapse or complete cessation of the program or behavior. Work with your client in advance to develop strategies for difficult times (e.g., what will he/she do on vacation or if he/she gets sick).

- contracts—behavioral contracts have been shown to enhance compliance. Be sure that the contract is written so that success is likely. Clients should feel reasonably confident that they can fulfill the contract.

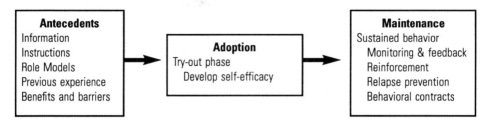

The Transtheoretical Model

The Transtheoretical Model also outlines stages of change. These stages are:

1. **Pre-contemplation**—People in this stage are not even thinking about a new behavior pattern (such as exercising). They are usually unmotivated, resistant, and engaged in avoidance tactics (e.g., if exercise comes up in conversation, they change the subject). They are clearly not ready for change and may even deny the need for change. Typically, pre-contemplaters tremendously underestimate the number of benefits of exercise, often citing only one or two when in actuality benefits number over 50. Instead, they may list many negatives (e.g., will get sweaty, have to buy new shoes, no time, might get injured, and will look silly). Since most American adults are sedentary[56] and appear to have little interest in exercising, a continuing challenge for the health/fitness professional lies in finding ways to move people out of this stage.

2. **Contemplation**—During this stage individuals are seriously considering change. They are more aware of the benefits but still aren't ready. They may talk about losing weight or starting an exercise program, but haven't taken any steps.

3. **Preparation**—Individuals in this stage are "preparing" to change by initially making small changes. They may call a health club, buy an exercise video, or even buy a piece of home exercise equipment. They usually intend to take action within a month or so.

4. **Action**—At this point, people are actively changing their behavior. As with the Adoption phase of the the Health Behavior Change Model, the first six weeks to six months is the most difficult period and the most common time to drop out.[57] Many clients initiating change are not really prepared for a six-month commitment; they think they'll achieve results much more quickly. Development of self-efficacy is critical, as is a supportive, motivating personal fitness trainer who provides realistic expectations.

5. **Maintenance**—This is the stage that sustains long-term, ongoing consciousness of the new behavior and successful integration of it into the lifestyle. (See strategies for enhancing maintenance, above.)[58]

The Transtheoretical Model is a continuum which holds that behavior change is not absolute, and that those who stop performing a given behavior may intend to start again (this holds true for both healthy or positive behaviors as well as for those that are unhealthy or negative).

What You Can Do To Support Behavior Change

1. **Emphasize benefits**—Educate clients about the 50+ benefits of exercise, the benefits of a heart-healthy diet, etc. Ask them what benefits they feel they're receiving. Remind them of their continued fitness progress, increased energy and better sleep. Most people feel much better at the end of an exercise session; help your clients to internalize this sense of well-being with a simple question, such as: "So, how do you feel now?" Help them develop an inner sense of satisfaction, and increase their intrinsic reward for behavior change.

2. **Set appropriate, achievable goals**—You may use the Goal Setting form in Appendix C, and/or use the SMART system of goal setting. SMART stands for Specific, Measurable, Action-oriented, Realistic, and Timed. Defined, specific goals are much easier to focus on than vague statements, such as: "I want to get in shape." Help your client define measurable, tangible goals, so that it will be clear when the goal has been achieved, and thus enhance motivation. Fitness assessments are ideal for establishing a base line and then giving proof of progress at later re-evaluations. Structure at least one goal so that you will be able to measure progress during reassessment. Action-oriented goal setting means writing out the details of the plan including: the days, times, duration and intensity. Realistic goals are critical for ensuring the success of your client. A timed goal is one with a target date for reassessment. Having a target date gives your client something to work toward and provides additional focus. In general, short-term goals of two to four weeks are more effective than long-term goals. Adjust goals frequently depending on the client's progress and needs.

3. **Avoid giving "too much, too soon"**—This is the major cause of injury and drop-out with new exercisers. When beginners exercise five or more days per week, and/or for longer than 45 minutes at a time, and/or at intensities greater than 85% of max VO_2, studies show increased injury rates and decreased compliance with the exercise program.[29] Instead, utilize the behavioral principle of shaping, or

progression. This is the concept of slow, steady, gradual, one-step-at-a-time improvement. When applying the principle of overload, it's best to do so conservatively, especially with beginner exercisers.

4. **Provide rewards and reinforcement**—This is said to be the most effective method for changing behavior. Let the client have a say in what type of reward works best for him/her: e.g., praise, certificates, headbands, and public recognition (as in an incentive contest, such as Travel Across America or Member of the Month). A fitness reassessment documenting positive change can also be a motivating reinforcer.

5. **Give feedback**—This can also be a formalized fitness reassessment, or it can be as simple as day-to-day reminders of progress. Pointing out to your client that he/she is able to lift more weight or walk faster than was possible two weeks ago provides continuing reassurance of progress. Documentation in the form of an exercise record or log is essential for tracking accomplishments.

6. **Prepare your client for potential setbacks**—Find out what kinds of obstacles your client might face and discuss strategies for difficult times. Vacations, holidays, family obligations and work pressures may all be cause for a temporary lapse. Help the client understand that this is normal; however, the goal is to persevere and not let the lapse turn into a "collapse" or a cessation of the behavior.

7. **Help the client use reminders**—Reminders are environmental cues, or prompts, that are used at home, in the car and at the workplace, to name a few, which help remind or provide a stimulus to exercise (or continue the desired behavior). Examples include: setting out exercise clothes the night before, always carrying exercise shoes in the car, writing exercise times into an appointment book, having a timer go off when it's time to exercise, placing post-it notes on the refrigerator, and always exercising with a buddy.

8. **Use behavioral contracts**—Contracts have been found to enhance success in 12-step programs. They help clients accept self-responsibility for their behavior as well as provide a time frame and focus for their goals. Many contracts include a reward for goal accomplishment and involve a significant other (as a witness). Be sure the goal is realistic and achievable (see "Behavior Contract" in Appendix B).

9. **Help "generalize" behavior**—This means that the clients don't only practice the new behavior (such as exercise) when they're with you. Provide them with alternatives for home exercise and exercise when traveling or on vacation. Develop your clients' confidence so they can continue the behavior on their own. Help clients incorporate increased activity into their daily lives and not to regard exercise as always having to be programmed and routine.

10. **Prevent boredom**—Many people view exercise as boring and unpleasant. Devise strategies that work for each client that help make exercise fun, motivating and interesting. This may mean crosstraining, taking indoor exercise outside and vice versa, or exercising with a friend. Recognize that the sheer repetitiveness of cardiorespiratory exercise (such as treadmill walking or stair-climbing) is boring for most. If possible, encourage reading, watching TV, listening to music, or some other distraction to help clients stick with it.

11. **Be a good role model**—Practicing what you preach in terms of exercise, healthy eating habits, positive body image, not smoking, and disease and disability prevention (such as proper lifting to prevent future back problems) provides an incentive for clients who see that a healthy and fit lifestyle is possible.

Communication Skills

Personal fitness trainers should constantly strive to improve their communication skills. Clear communication reduces both personal stress and the stress felt by those around you. It helps you be a more effective, inspiring leader. It also helps you understand your client better and allows you to work together to create the best program for optimal results.

To create client trust and confidence, you must establish a sense of support, a sense that you are really there for that client. This is especially important at the first meeting. Three qualities that are useful for creating supportive relationships by those in the helping professions are empathy, warmth, and genuineness.[59]

■ Being **empathetic** means putting yourself in your clients' shoes and really seeing their point of view. It means being open and receptive to your clients.

■ Being **warm** is exemplified by a spirit of friendliness and openness that is non-judgmental. Giving clients your understanding and undivided attention helps them to open up, feel safe, and foster self-acceptance.

■ Being **genuine** is simply letting your deep sense of caring come through. Think back to why you wanted to become a personal trainer. Let your spirit of earnestness and honesty be there for your clients.

Active, conscious listening

Giving full support to clients demands your full attention. Being a good listener helps your clients to feel valued, understood and truly heard. Here are some steps toward active listening:

■ Use open body language. Breathe deeply and allow your body to relax. Face your client and angle your body slightly toward him/her. Sit at the client's eye level and keep arms and legs uncrossed.

■ Maintain eye contact; a relaxed focus on your client without constantly shifting your eyes helps him/her to feel safe.

■ Remind yourself that your client is worthy of respect and attention.

■ Take the time to really listen. Be patient.

■ Drop expectations and fears about what you're going to do.

■ Use encouraging phrases that tell the client you're really listening and want to hear more (e.g., "I see," "Really," "Mmm, hmm").

■ Minimize distractions. Find a place where you won't be interrupted by other members, phone calls, etc.

Roadblocks to active listening

■ Comparing, always assessing, always noticing who is more fit, smart, emotionally healthy, or who has suffered more, etc.—You won't really hear or understand your client if your thoughts always come back to yourself.

■ Rehearsing—If you're always busy planning what you'll say next, or what story you'll tell, you won't really hear your client.

■ Filtering, or listening to some things but not to others–Letting your mind wander or avoiding hearing certain things (such as negative or critical statements) will prevent you from completely hearing what the client is saying.

■ Judging—Labeling someone as stupid, crazy or any other negative term means you've stopped listening and are having a "knee jerk" reaction.

■ Blaming or criticizing—This tends to shame the client, creating a loss of self-confidence.

- Being right—If you always have to be right, you may go to any lengths to avoid being wrong (twisting the facts, making excuses, etc.).

- Dreaming, half-listening—If you tend to dream often when others are talking, you may be bored or anxious. Reconsider your commitment to really knowing your clients and valuing what they have to say.

- Identifying—Here again, the focus has more to do with you than with your client. In this case, everything the client says reminds you of something you've felt, done or suffered. You're so busy thinking about your life that you don't really hear your client.

- Advising—Even though you are being paid to support, help, and advise, be sure you fully listen before jumping in with suggestions. Some trainers only hear a sentence or two before they start trying to problem-solve, often missing what's really important in the process.

- Derailing—Suddenly changing the subject or "joking it off" causes you to avoid seriously listening to your client.

- Placating—Wanting others to like you, you just go along with whatever is said. You agree without really hearing.

- Minimizing—Telling clients not to worry, or that their particular problem isn't so bad, lessens the importance of the message.

- Denying—Implying that clients don't have a problem when they feel they do, makes them feel as if they haven't been heard or understood.

Supporting through verbal responses

Giving appropriate verbal responses that encourage your client to keep talking is a form of active listening. Some techniques include:

- Mirror—Restate the client's message.

- Paraphrase—Put the core of the client's message into your own words for greater clarity.

- Ask for clarification of a client's statements.

- Search for more information. Use open-ended questions (see below).

- Acknowledge—Give the client direct feedback about what you hear the client saying. This is better accepted if your statements begin with "I" or another personal pronoun (e.g., "I hear that you're not feeling well today").

- Summarize—Recap what was said and never let a conversation end without being sure of what was said and why. Don't pretend to understand if you don't.

Using open- and close-ended questions

The use of open-ended questions encourages more conversation and disclosure of information.[60] This is ideal when you are trying to really understand a client. Open-ended questions:

■ invite a free-flowing answer

■ open up conversations

■ usually start with words like how, what, why, could or would

Examples of open-ended questions are: "Would you tell me about your goals?" "What would you like to get out of our session today?" "How do you think you can best improve your health?"

Close-ended questions may be used to gain facts and narrow the discussion. Closed-ended questions:

■ can be answered in a few words

■ close off discussion

■ give the questioner control of the conversation

■ direct the discussion

■ limit the kind of information obtained

Examples of closed-ended questions are: "How old are you?" "Do you like weight training?"

Clearer communication through "I" statements

Owning your thoughts and feelings helps you gain personal control of yourself, both in professional and personal interactions. Statements that use such words as "it," "you," "people," "they," and "we" place responsibility on someone or something else besides yourself. Some examples:

"It is strange talking to you" instead of "I feel strange talking to you."

"People feel nervous in new situations" instead of "I feel nervous in new situations."

"We should end the session now" instead of "I think it's time to end the session."

Avoid the use of qualifiers and nullifiers. Qualifiers are ways of watering down the truth; nullifiers help avoid or escape the truth. Both decrease self-responsibility. Examples of qualifiers include: "I guess," "I suppose," "perhaps," "maybe," "kind of," "probably," "only," "just," and "sort of." Examples of nullifiers include: "I should" instead of "I could" "I can't" instead of "I won't;" and "I don't know" instead of "I don't care to find out."

Motivating your clients with appropriate verbal cues

What you say while your clients are plugging away on the treadmill or performing their sets and repetitions can make all the difference. Good cueing is specific (what exactly is correct and what needs improvement), provides the information necessary for correction, and is worded positively. Negative cueing uses words such as "don't", "try", "can't", "difficult", "doubt" and "ought to". These words have been shown to decrease motivation and positive feelings.[61] A positive cue helps the client by suggesting what to do instead of what not to do. For example: "Keep your abdominals tight throughout the lift" is more effective than "Don't let your belly hang out, or your back arch." When you cue in a positive manner, you use the client's name frequently and recognize his/her effort. Your body language and verbal cues should be congruent for maximum effectiveness, which means that what you say matches your body signals. (Looking distractedly around the room while praising your client sends a mixed message.)

Inspire and help your clients to believe in themselves by using affirmations and promoting a positive attitude and self-acceptance. You may affirm a positive quality in someone by stating a quality that he/she currently possesses or is capable of attaining in the near future. Always word the affirmation as if it were a fact now, in the present. For example: "Susan, you are really powerful when you do those push-ups." "Paul, you are certainly full of energy!" "Liz, you are consistent and dedicated."

Clients that come to you with little knowledge and low motivation will need a high level of support and direction. As the relationship evolves and the client develops feelings of self-efficacy and confidence, less hand-holding will be necessary. You will know you are truly successful when your client has fully adopted a healthy lifestyle and achieved long-term adherence when they exercise and eat right because they want to. Their sense of inner satisfaction is their ongoing motivator; their good health habits are their own immediate reward. Once a client has reached such a level of self-motivation he/she may no longer need your professional support and guidance, however, you'll know you have achieved the ultimate success as an educator and a motivator of people.

IN SUMMARY

In this chapter, two important models for behavior change were discussed: the Health Behavior Change Model and the Transtheoretical Model. Eleven practical strategies were listed to help clients with lifestyle changes. Basic communication skills were introduced, including: active listening, blocks to listening, supportive verbal responses, open-ended questions, and the use of "I" statements.

Chapter **9**

Special Populations

Low Back

As stated earlier, low back pain is a common problem, afflicting 80% of adults at some point in their lives.[6] A major factor in preventable back pain is poor body mechanics, how an individual sits, stands, walks, sleeps, lifts and exercises as well as performs activities of daily living. It is difficult to have proper body mechanics if important major muscles are weak and/or tight. Common postural imbalances that contribute to back pain are excessive lordosis (swayback) and excessive kyphosis (hunchback); these imbalances often result from muscles that are too tight and/or too weak. Other risk factors for low back pain are: loss of flexibility and muscle endurance, loss of torso stabilization, poor posture, excessive forward flexion, and poor cardiovascular fitness. Loosely linked to the development of low back pain (LBP) are: high mental stress or inadequate coping mechanisms, obesity and smoking.[62]

In order to provide safe, effective and appropriate exercises for your clients, it is important to first understand the basic anatomy of the spine.

Quick Anatomy Review

There are approximately 32 vertebrae in the spine, divided into cervical (7), thoracic (12), lumbar (5), sacral (5), and coccygeal (2-4 fused) regions. When the spine is in neutral alignment it should have four curves: a lordotic curve in the cervical region, a kyphotic curve in the thoracic region, a lordotic curve in the lumbar spine, and a kyphotic curve in the sacral spine. Each vertebrae has an opening through which the spinal cord passes (the foramen) and several protrusions, or processes. There are two sets of articulations: between the vertebral bodies (and disks), and between the facet joints. Disks have two parts: the outer fibers (annulus fibrosus) and the inner core (nucleus pulposus). Disks act as shock absorbers and permit compression and movement in several directions. Two long ligaments (anterior and posterior longitudinal ligaments) hold the vertebrae in place, top to bottom. The major muscles that support the spine are the: rectus abdominis and obliques, transverse abdominis, and erector spinae (including the longissimus, spinalis, iliocostalis and multifidus groups).

Excessive **lordosis** is characterized by an increased lumbosacral angle, increased lumbar lordosis, increased anterior pelvic tilt, and hip flexion.[63] It may be triggered by obesity, pregnancy, weak abdominal muscles, and poor body awareness. This typically causes pain by: stressing the anterior longitudinal ligament, narrowing the posterior disk space, compressing the related nerve root, causing the facet joints to become weight bearing, resulting in muscle strains. Typical muscle imbalances that need to be corrected include:

- tight iliopsoas (hip flexors) that need to be stretched

- tight (and possibly weak) erector spinae that need to be stretched

- weak rectus abdominis, obliques and transversus that need to be strengthened

Tight hamstrings (that need to be stretched) are very common in the general public and can be a contributor to low back pain because they inhibit proper body mechanics. For example, it is more difficult to lift objects correctly and/or sit properly with shortened hamstring muscles.

The key is to teach prevention. For instance, show clients how to lift correctly, how to sit properly for long periods, how to sleep with minimal low back stress, how to rake leaves and shovel snow, and what risky exercises to avoid.

Excessive **kyphosis** (hunchback/rounded shoulders) is characterized by an increased thoracic curve, abducted scapulae, and often an accompanying forward head. Pain may be caused by stress to the posterior longitudinal ligament and fatigue of the thoracic erector spinae, mid-trapezius and rhomboid muscles. Major muscle imbalances that may need to be corrected include:

- tight pectoralis major, pectoralis minor, and serratus anterior

- tight anterior deltoid

- tight latissimus dorsi

- tight levator scapulae and upper trapezius

- weak, overstretched scapular adductors: mid-trapezius and rhomboids

Stretch the tight muscles and strengthen the weak muscles. Avoid an over emphasis on shoulder flexion work. Help clients to be aware of the forward head (chin jut) posture which often accompanies kyphosis and is easy to fall into when fatigued.

Scoliosis is a sideways or lateral curvature of the spine. Since this postural misalignment is often congenital and may have serious consequences (especially for developing children), a diagnosis should be made by a medical professional and corrective exercises should be prescribed by a physical therapist.

Pregnancy

Most pregnant women can and should exercise. However, all pregnant clients should have clearances from their physicians prior to training. Pregnancy causes profound changes in a woman's body, including:

■ connective tissue changes resulting in an enlarged pelvis, ligament laxity and joint instability

■ changes in center of gravity due to enlarging uterus and breasts

■ increased lordosis and strain on the sacroiliac and hip joints resulting in increased potential for back pain and risk of falls

■ nerve compression syndromes, such as carpal tunnel syndrome due to increased fluid retention

■ total blood volume increase (30–50% increase over pre-pregnancy levels) with the major increase coming from plasma volume

■ increased heart rate, cardiac output and blood pressure both at rest and during exercise

■ potential compression of the vena cava by the enlarging uterus (especially in the supine position)

■ displacement of the diaphragm upward, potentially causing discomfort and shortness of breath

■ lateral expansion of the rib cage

■ increased need for calories (~ 300 additional calories per day[64])

■ increased basal metabolic rate

■ increased heat production and decreased tolerance of heat

■ increased fatigue and nauseousness (especially in first trimester)

■ diastasis recti (split in the rectus abdominis)

■ tendency toward constipation and heartburn

■ tendency toward varicosities in legs and pelvic area

■ difficulty sleeping

■ fluctuating emotions

There are several benefits of exercise during pregnancy. These include: improved circulation, improved digestion and elimination, improved muscle tone to support joints, increased energy and endurance, better ability to regulate body temperature, improved posture, improved body image and self-esteem, relief of discomforts, such as backaches, leg cramps, and fatigue, improved support of pelvic organs with pelvic floor strengthening, decreased stress, improved sleep, increased control of excessive weight gain, and possible sense of control during labor. Keep in mind, however, that there is little to no research supporting claims that exercise ensures a shorter, less painful labor, or that babies born to exercising mothers are healthier than those born to non-exercisers.

Because it is extremely important not to compromise fetal or maternal well-being, there are some concerns regarding prenatal exercise.

- Strenuous exercisers may gain less weight and deliver lighter babies than sedentary women.[65] Under conditions of hard labor, nutritional stress, and prolonged standing, strenuous exercise has been shown to adversely affect fetal growth.[66]

- There is concern that exercise may result in elevated body temperature to a degree that would cause negative effects on the fetus (especially to the sensitive neural cells). This has been shown in animal studies; and women exposed to heat in the first trimester (hot tubs, saunas, and fevers) have shown an increase in fetal neural tube defects.[67] However, there are no human studies showing that exercise can elevate core body temperature to the extent that the fetus would be affected. Most experts recommend that core temperature not exceed 38°C, or 101°F.

- Shunting of blood to the working muscles during exercise decreases utero-placental blood flow and may compromise fetal oxygen supply. In animal studies, this has resulted in altered fetal growth.

- There is a concern that exercising muscles will compete with the fetus for glucose. During pregnancy, carbohydrates are utilized at a greater rate during exercise, and fluctuations in glucose levels are larger, both of which may put the mother and the fetus at greater risk of hypoglycemia (carbohydrate stores are the fetus' primary energy source for growth and development). Repeated hypoglycemic episodes may inhibit fetal growth.[68]

The 1994 American College of Obstetricians and Gynecologists (ACOG) Guidelines for Exercise During Pregnancy

1. Regular exercise (at least three times per week) is preferable to intermittent activity.

2. Avoid exercise in the supine position after the first trimester. Avoid prolonged periods of motionless standing.

3. Modify exercise intensity according to symptoms. Stop exercising when fatigued and do not exercise to exhaustion. Non-weight bearing exercise may be preferable.

4. Avoid exercises where there is a significant potential for loss of balance or abdominal trauma.

5. Exercising pregnant women should be especially careful to consume an adequate diet.

6. Ensure adequate hydration, wear appropriate clothing, and strive for optimal environmental surroundings during exercise to help dissipate heat (especially in the first trimester).

7. Resume pre-pregnancy routines gradually postpartum.[142]

Other recommendations addressing exercise and pregnancy include:

1. Know the absolute and relative contraindications to exercise during pregnancy as well as pregnancy danger signs (available from ACOG as well as in the AFAA Prenatal Fitness Home Study and Workshop Manuals).

2. Use RPE to help determine proper intensity.

3. Sedentary pregnant women should not begin an exercise program in the first or third trimesters.

4. Perform push-ups in a standing position against the wall after the first trimester.

5. Weight training may be continued throughout pregnancy if the client has used weights regularly before, utilizes spotters when necessary, avoids maximal lifts, and has medical clearance to weight train.

6. Abdominal exercise is indicated for most pregnant clients as long as there is no Valsalva maneuver and as long as a position other than supine is used (side-lying, standing, or all fours are acceptable). Check for diastasis (a split in the rectus abdominis) by having the client lie supine with knees bent (this only takes a few seconds), and curl up. If there is a diastasis, it will be near the navel, and will be vertically oriented. Assess the width of the split with fingertips (determine if it is one, two or three finger widths wide). If the client has a separation, curl-ups should be performed while splinting the gap with the hands (this applies primarily to women in the first trimester and/or who are postpartum). No oblique work should be

performed with a diastasis, and regular curl-ups should be avoided if the separation is greater than three fingers in width.

7. Pelvic floor exercises (Kegels) should be performed regularly.

8. All stretching exercises should be static.

9. Pregnancy is a time to maintain fitness, not strive for dramatic improvements.

Seniors

According to the U.S. Bureau of the Census (1996), the population of people over the age of 64 in the U.S. will increase by 14% over the next 10 years. This represents a significant marketing niche for personal fitness trainers. Although there is a wide spectrum of ability and fitness levels among the elderly, there are a number of common characteristics of aging that affect exercise programming, including:

- decreased maximal heart rate as a result of increased "stiffness" of the ventricular walls and slower ventricle filling (stroke volume also declines, leading to a reduced cardiac output)
- decreased VO_2 max (about 9% per decade in inactive men, and about 5% per decade in active men)[70], largely due to the reduced cardiac output
- increasing blood pressure, primarily resulting from progressive atherosclerosis
- increased use of medications, especially those for hypertension and cardiac arrhythmias (there is an increased likelihood of underlying coronary artery disease in older clients)
- slower reaction time due to a slower velocity of nerve conduction (slows by about 10–15% by age 70)
- progressive loss of bone mass (osteoporosis) and bone strength, especially in women, and the degeneration of joint cartilage causing an increase in osteoarthritis, which then increases the likelihood of back and knee problems
- decreasing lean body mass (with a related decrease in muscle strength and power) and increasing percentage of body fat (creeping obesity) which is partly due to a slowing of the BMR (~ 2% per decade), as well as to increasing inactivity
- declining flexibility, particularly in the inactive, due to connective tissue changes in the muscles, ligaments, joint capsules, and tendons
- increased tendency toward dehydration due to decline in kidney function
- increased susceptibility to soreness and injury

There are many benefits of exercise for seniors, including: increased strength with mild to moderate muscle hypertrophy, increased bone density, improvements in joint range of motion, improved balance, increased VO_2 max, increased lean body mass, decreased percentage of body fat, improved glucose tolerance, improved cholesterol status, decreased stress, enhanced sense of well-being, and improved ability to carry out activities of daily living.

Guidelines for senior programming

1. Obtain a medical history and a physician's clearance prior to fitness testing and/or exercise.

2. Recognize individual differences in senior fitness levels.

3. Remember that too much, too soon is the major cause of injury and drop-out. Focus on safety with clients. Remember that many elderly are afraid they might overdo or become sore.

4. Include a longer warm-up and cool-down.

5. Consider minimal or non-weight bearing activities, such as cycling, swimming, and water, chair and floor exercises for clients with significant musculoskeletal limitations.

6. If arthritis flares up, reduce the intensity and duration of the workout. When arthritic joints are pain-free, concentrate on gentle range of motion type movements.

7. Emphasize functional exercises (those that relate to activities of daily living), such as walking, stair-climbing and squats, whenever possible. Help clients maintain their ability to pick up grandchildren, garden, button clothing, open cans, and so on. Balance and coordination exercises are also beneficial for improved self-care.

8. Moderate strength training is appropriate for clients without orthopedic problems. Keep repetitions slow and controlled.

9. Emphasize flexibility work to help maintain joint range of motion. Mobility exercises for hands, wrists and feet may be important.

10. If the client has had a recent graded exercise stress test, consult with the physician and/or exercise test technologist to determine appropriate cardiovascular intensity (this is especially important for clients with CAD). Use the RPE method to assess intensity if the client is on blood pressure or cardiac medication.

11. The longer a client has been sedentary and/or the more limitations he/she has, the lower the starting intensity.

12. Be alert for signs of joint pain, distress or overtraining.

13. Help build your client's confidence in his/her ability to exercise safely and enjoyably. Encourage long-term maintenance of the exercise habit.

Hypertension

Hypertension is a common health problem, afflicting one in four Americans and, as a subgroup, one in three African Americans.[1,17] It is a major risk factor for the development of heart disease, stroke, kidney failure, and congestive heart failure. Although the tendency for hypertension may be inherited, everyday health habits strongly affect the development of high blood pressure. Lifestyle factors influencing blood pressure include:

- high sodium intake (⅓ of all hypertensives are sodium sensitive)
- high dietary saturated fat intake
- cigarette smoking
- heavy alcohol consumption
- obesity
- high stress lifestyle
- physical inactivity

Normal, or average, blood pressure is usually thought to be around 120/80 mm Hg. Both the ACSM and the AHA define high blood pressure as starting at 140/90 mm Hg (measured on at least two separate occasions), or on blood pressure medication. The top number is referred to as the systolic pressure, or the amount of pressure or force exerted against the arterial walls immediately after the heart has contracted. The bottom number, or diastolic pressure, may be thought of as the "run off" force, or the amount of pressure still remaining against the arterial walls as the heart relaxes before the next contraction.

Programming recommendations for hypertensives

1. Learn to take blood pressure measurements. Hypertensives should have their blood pressure monitored frequently (ideally before, during and after exercise). However, check with your state's laws regarding determination of vital signs. In some states, blood pressure may only be taken by a licensed health care provider.

2. Respect the limits of your expertise. There are some clients with hypertension and/or heart disease who need to be in a medically supervised program where emergency care is available. These clients may include: those whose systolic BP decreases with exercise; those who frequently have resting systolic BP >160 mm Hg or resting diastolic BP >90 mm Hg; and those with an abnormal increase in BP >200/100 mm Hg.

3. Be alert for symptoms of heart disease (see Chapter 2), onset of angina (chest pain), or an inappropriate drop in HR. Notify a physician promptly.

4. An intensity of 40–65% of max HR is recommended by the American Association of Cardiovascular and Pulmonary Rehabilitation.[71] Studies have shown that mild to moderate intensity exercise may be better than high intensity exercise at controlling hypertension.

5. Use the RPE method of assessing intensity if your client is on blood pressure medication.

6. Be familiar with the exercise effects of blood pressure medications. Consult the client's physician or pharmacologist when in doubt.

7. Use caution when recommending strength training to hypertensives. Avoid very heavy weights and clenched fists. Keep intensity low, and increase the number of repetitions. Avoid resistance training to the point of failure, even if weights are light.

8. Avoid isometric training due to the likelihood of straining with a closed throat (Valsalva maneuver), which may cause an elevation in blood pressure.

9. Avoid positions in which the feet are higher than the head.

10. Teach relaxation and stress management techniques.

Diabetes

Diabetes mellitus is a metabolic disease caused by problems with blood sugar utilization. Blood sugar, or glucose, is necessary for both anaerobic and aerobic metabolic pathways. Insulin helps make cell walls more permeable, and promotes the entry of the large glucose molecule into the cells, where it can be used for energy. There are two types of diabetes: Type I (juvenile onset), or IDDM (insulin dependent diabetes mellitus), and Type II (adult onset), or NIDDM (non-insulin dependent diabetes mellitus). IDDM diabetics usually depend on daily injections of insulin, as their pancreas does not produce enough, if any, insulin. NIDDM diabetics do manufacture insulin, but their cells have decreased insulin sensitivity, and so do not accept glucose inside. In both cases, hyperglycemia (high blood sugar) results. The majority (about 90%) of diabetics are NIDDM.

NIDDM diabetics may or may not need to take insulin, and may be able to manage their disease completely with diet and exercise. Exercise has an insulin-like effect, assisting the entry of glucose into the cells and enhancing insulin sensitivity. However, if exercise is excessive, or if the diet is inadequate, glucose levels may suddenly drop and the diabetic may become hypoglycemic. A hypoglycemic reaction (also known as insulin shock) is potentially life-threatening and you should help your client take steps for prevention, including:

1. Work with your client's physician (a medical clearance is essential). Insulin dosage should be appropriate for an exercising diabetic.

2. Keep the emergency medical number and your emergency response plan handy.

3. For one hour after injection, avoid exercising muscles that have been injected.

4. Do not exercise at the time of peak insulin action.

5. Have your client eat carbohydrate snacks before and during prolonged exercise, unless directed otherwise by his/her physician.

6. Always have some form of sugar available and help client to stay hydrated.

7. Monitor blood glucose frequently, especially when starting a program.

8. Know the signs of hypoglycemia, including: excessive fatigue, nausea, lightheadedness, dizziness, spots in front of eyes, confusion, shakiness, headaches, sudden rapid heart rate, and even seizures.

Other recommendations include:

■ Promote aerobic exercise. Cardiovascular exercise is ideal for diabetics because it helps with weight control, increases insulin sensitivity, and increases glucose tolerance. Regular, consistent steady-state exercise at the same time each day is best for helping to control diabetes.

■ Help clients practice good foot hygiene. One outcome of diabetes is nerve damage and accelerated atherosclerosis (resulting in poor circulation) in the extremities. Sores, blisters and cuts may become infected and gangrenous without the clients' knowledge, since they may have reduced sensation in their feet.

IN SUMMARY

In this chapter, low back risk factors, anatomy, terminology, and client recommendations were briefly covered. Physiological changes during pregnancy, exercise benefits, concerns, and guidelines for exercise during pregnancy were discussed. Characteristics of aging, exercise benefits, and guidelines for senior programming were explored.

Lifestyle factors that influence hypertension and exercise programming for those with high blood pressure were reviewed. Finally, basic guidelines for working with diabetics were explained.

Chapter 10

Weightroom Skills and Exercises

Proper Lifting and Spotting Techniques

Proper lifting technique is one of the most important skills you can teach your client. Lifting is a functional activity of daily living, and when done improperly, can lead to back pain or other serious injury. Points to remember when lifting a bar:

- Use the correct grip. Always use a closed (thumbs wrapped around the bar) grip. Grips may be underhand (supinated), overhand (pronated), or alternate (mixed). Be sure to place hands on the bar so that it is balanced. Grip width on the bar may be shoulder-width apart (common), narrow, or wide.

- Position the body correctly. Feet should be far enough apart that the body has an adequate base of support and is balanced (usually shoulder-width apart). Knees and feet should be aligned in the same direction. When lowering the body to grasp the bar, heels need to stay in contact with the floor, and hips need to press backwards and stay low. Practice hip flexion, not spinal flexion on the descent. Hips should be in an anterior pelvic tilt and the natural curvature of the spine should be maintained. Do not drop hips below knee level as this stresses knee ligaments and tendons. Scapulae are adducted, head is up, and eyes look straight ahead.

- Tighten the abdominals and keep the bar close when lifting. Use the leg muscles, not the back, and straighten to full extension of the hips and knees (avoid hyperextension). Exhale as the knees extend.

■ When lifting bar up to shoulders, keep the upward movement of the bar smooth and continuous. Do not let the bar rest on the thighs. As the knees and hips extend, flex the elbows, abduct the shoulders, keep wrists as neutral as possible, and "rack" the bar in front of the shoulders. If the bar is heavy, it may be necessary to rise up on the balls of the feet as legs straighten, elevate the scapulae when abducting the shoulders, and flex the knees slightly when the bar makes contact with the collarbone.

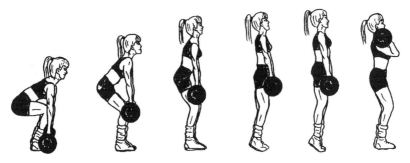

Fig. 10.1–Correct lifting with barbell

As a client's personal fitness trainer, one of your paid (and legal) responsibilities is to provide proper spotting to the client. High risk exercises, such as barbell squats, bench presses and incline presses demand particular awareness. Failures to spot, under some circumstances (in at least one case), has been judged to be tantamount to willful and wanton conduct. As a consequence, it is very important for you to adhere to safe spotting guidelines for your clients. Follow these general guidelines for spotting:

General Spotting Guidelines

■ It is your responsibility to keep loose plates, barbells, dumbbells, and other equipment in their place and out of your client's way.

■ Be sure that you are strong enough to assist your client if needed. Some exercises, such as a back squat, may need more than one spotter.

■ Practice prevention. When spotting, keep your knees flexed, back in neutral alignment, and abdominals tight in case you have to suddenly assist.

■ Keep hands as close to the bar as possible without obstructing the movement of the bar. When assisting, use the appropriate closed grip for the lift.

■ Make sure the bar is evenly loaded; always use collars or clips.

■ Communicate with your client about how many more repetitions will be performed and whether or not you are going to assist.

■ Assist any time the predetermined movement speed decreases.

Specific guidelines for spotting will be included for the individual exercises that follow.

Teaching Method for Proper Exercise Technique

How do you teach clients new exercises and/or refine their performance on exercises they already know? The whole-part-whole, and the demo-detail-demo methods of teaching are modified below. This method will help you give clear, specific instructions and will help sharpen your awareness of proper technique.

Step 1: Identify:

- name of exercise
- equipment used
- major muscles worked

Step 2: Demonstrate the exercise (show the "whole" movement)

Step 3: Give specific details about the exercise (break down the "parts")

- show the starting position including the grip and grip width
- discuss which joints are stabilized and which joints should move
- explain proper alignment and technique
- teach clients to consciously contract, or "engage," the muscle
- go over safety and injury factors; discuss common errors

Step 4: Demonstrate the exercise again ("whole")

Some personal fitness trainers recommend having the client repeat all four steps themselves to help integrate the information (especially when learning a new exercise). Another useful technique is visualization; have your client visualize the entire exercise before lifting.

Teaching Specific Weightroom Exercises

The remainder of this Chapter is designed to help you make sense of common exercises: the muscles involved, their line of pull, proper form and technique, spotting guidelines (when appropriate), and common errors. For further clarification of joint actions and terminology, see Chapter 5, Kinesiology Review. For basic strength training principles and recommendations, see Chapter 6, Muscular Strength, Endurance, and Flexibility Programming. Keep in mind that joint actions always describe the concentric phase.

▼ Chest Exercises ▼

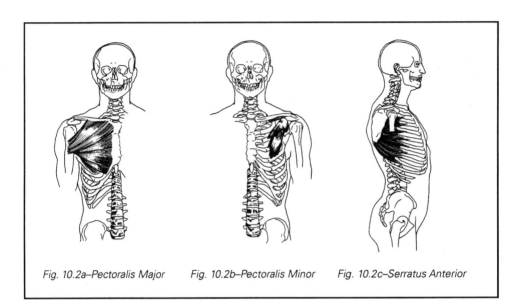

Fig. 10.2a–Pectoralis Major   Fig. 10.2b–Pectoralis Minor   Fig. 10.2c–Serratus Anterior

Muscle	Prime Mover for:	Assists with:
Pectoralis Major	shoulder flexion (clavicular portion) shoulder horizontal flexion (both parts) shoulder adduction (sternal portion) shoulder extension (sternal portion)	shoulder internal rotation
Pectoralis Minor	scapular depression scapular abduction scapular downward rotation	
Serratus Anterior	scapular abduction scapular upward rotation	

Bench Press

Equipment used: barbell or dumbbells, flat bench

Moving joints	Joint action	Muscles worked
shoulders	horizontal flexion	pectoralis major, anterior deltoid, coracobrachialis
elbows	extension	triceps
Optional: shoulder girdle	abduction	pectoralis minor, serratus anterior

1. Starting position: Lie supine, feet flat on floor or on bench, back is in neutral, pelvis is posteriorly tilted. Use wide, closed, pronated grip (narrow grip = greater triceps involvement) with evenly spaced hands.

2. Moving joints: Shoulders and elbows move. All other joints should be stabilized, including the scapulae, unless pec minor and serratus anterior strengthening is a goal, in which case abduct the scapulae at the end of the shoulder/elbow range of motion. Keep spine and wrists stabilized.

3. Alignment and technique: Upper arm is angled 80°–90° out from torso; forearms are perpendicular to floor. Exhale on the upward phase, inhale on the downward phase.

4. Engage and contract the pecs, anterior deltoids, and triceps.

5. Safety factors: Movement of bar is slow and controlled; watch for uncontrolled descent and avoid extreme end range of motion in order to decrease shoulder joint stress. Have client let you know when he/she's performing the final repetition. Watch for wrists rolling, back arching, hips pressing up, bouncing the bar off the sternum. Many exercisers attempt to lift too much weight to maintain proper form. Use three spotters for heavy loads.

Spotting guidelines: Assist with unracking and racking the bar. Stand behind bench with flexed knees and neutral spine (abdominals in). Use alternate grip inside the client's hands and spot the bar on both descent and ascent.

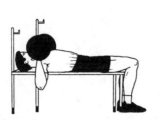 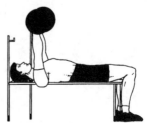

Fig. 10.3–Flat barbell bench press

Incline Press, Decline Press

Equipment used: barbell or dumbbells, incline bench or decline bench

The moving joints, working muscles, and joint actions are akin to those used in the standard flat bench press (on previous page). However, keep in mind the following information.

Incline press

- Due to the increasingly vertical line of pull (depending on the incline), the clavicular fibers of the pectoralis major are targeted.

- The greater the incline, the greater the anterior and medial deltoid involvement (the shoulder joint action becomes more like abduction).

- The greater the incline, the greater the tendency to elevate the shoulder girdle and involve the upper trapezius fibers, as well as the levator scapulae and rhomboids (responsible for elevation). See training tips under shoulder military (overhead) press.

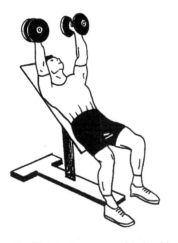
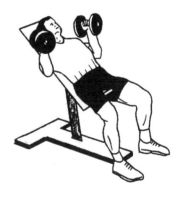

Fig. 10.4–Incline press with dumbbells

Decline press

- With the head lower than the chest, the sternal fibers of the pectoralis major are emphasized.

- The greater the decline, the more the shoulder joint movement becomes like adduction. Prime movers for adduction are the latissimus dorsi, teres major, and sternal portion of the pecs.

- Depending on client goals, there is an opportunity for resisted shoulder girdle depression at the end of the range of motion. This would utilize the pectoralis minor and the lower trapezius fibers.

Starting position, moving and stabilized joints, alignment, safety factors, and spotting guidelines are all similar to those for the bench press.

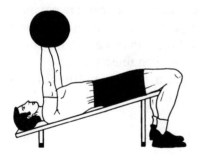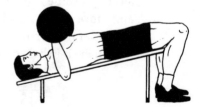

Fig. 10.5–Decline press with barbell

Dumbbell Fly (flat, incline or decline)

This exercise provides more isolation for the pectorals than the bench press since the elbows are held stable and the triceps are not involved (except as stabilizers).

Equipment used: dumbbells and flat, incline, or decline bench

Moving joints	Joint action	Muscles worked
shoulders	horizontal flexion	pectoralis major, anterior deltoid, coracobrachialis
Optional: shoulder girdle shoulders	abduction internal rotation	pectoralis minor, serratus anterior subscapularis, teres major

1. Starting position: Lie supine, feet flat on floor or on bench, back in neutral, pelvis posteriorly tilted. Start in up position, elbows slightly flexed, palms facing each other (mid pronated).

2. Moving joints: Shoulders move. Stabilize elbows, wrists, spine and pelvis. Scapulae should be stabilized unless pec minor and serratus anterior strengthening is a goal, in which case abduct the scapulae at the end of the shoulder range of motion.

3. Alignment and technique: Lower until upper arms are parallel with chest, keeping elbows in slightly flexed, stable position. Palms face up, although some trainers prefer to horizontally abduct the shoulders and move into external rotation, and then finish the movement with shoulders internally rotated (minimizing radio-ulnar joint movement). Exhale on upward phase.

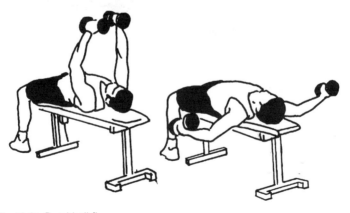

Fig. 10.6a–Dumbbell fly

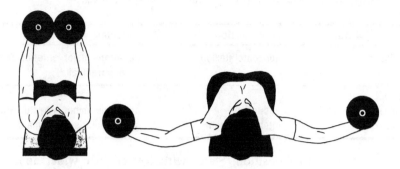

Fig. 10.6b–Dumbbell fly

4. Engage and contract the pecs and anterior deltoids. Keep the contraction throughout both the concentric and the eccentric phases.

5. Safety factors: Some professionals place this exercise on their "high risk" list because of the potential for an out-of-control descent and excessive range of motion, leading to shoulder injuries. Watch for problems with wrist breaking and elevated shoulders as well.

Spotting guidelines: Kneel or stand behind client's head and spot the forearms, wrists or dumbbells.

Bilateral Cable Cross-over

Equipment used: high pulleys, cable cross-over set-up

Moving joints	Joint action	Muscles worked
shoulders	horizontal flexion	pectoralis major, anterior deltoid, coracobrachialis
Optional: shoulder girdle shoulders	abduction internal rotation	pectoralis minor, serratus anterior subscapularis, teres major

1. Starting position: Stand with feet slightly wider apart than hip-width, or feet can be staggered. Knees are flexed, abdominals contracted, scapulae depressed and adducted, elbows slightly flexed. Start in the open position.

2. Moving joints: Shoulders move. Stabilize elbows and wrists. Pay particular attention to maintaining a neutral, stable position with the torso. Depress and stabilize scapulae unless pec minor and serratus anterior strengthening is a goal.

3. Alignment and technique: Exhale as arms are brought forward in horizontal plane. Internally rotate shoulders so that at full concentric contraction the thumbs are touching and palms are pronated (hands may also cross).

4. Engage and contract the pectoralis major and the anterior deltoids.

5. Safety factors: Too much weight can make this exercise very difficult to control. The potential for excessive range of motion and too much speed on the eccentric phase increases shoulder joint risk. Perform the eccentric phase slowly and keep shoulders and scapulae down.

Spotting guidelines: Stand in back of client and spot wrists/forearms.

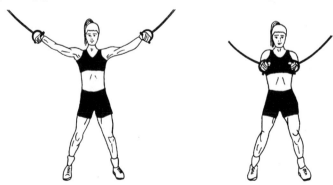

Fig. 10.7–Bilateral cable cross-over

Push-up

Optional equipment used: mat, aerobic (low) step, bench, wall

Moving joints	Joint action	Muscles worked
shoulders	horizontal flexion	pectoralis major, anterior deltoid, coracobrachialis
elbows	extension	triceps

Note: Muscles that work strongly as stabilizers (due to anti-gravity position) are the abdominals, erector spinae, gluteus maximus, trapezius, rhomboids, serratus anterior and pectoralis minor.

1. Starting position for flat (hands-on-floor) push-up: Distribute body weight on hands and knees or hands and toes. Start in up position. Neck, spine and pelvis in neutral position. For standard push-up, hands are slightly wider than shoulder-width apart with fingers facing straight ahead.

2. Moving joints: Shoulders and elbows move. Stabilization of all other joints is very important for injury prevention. There should be no movement of the spine, neck or pelvis.

3. Alignment and technique: Perform the exercise smoothly and avoid sagging through the back. Avoid hyperextending the elbows on the way up. Exhale on the way up, inhale down. Avoid looking up as this stresses the cervical vertebrae.

4. Engage and contract the pecs, anterior deltoids and the triceps.

5. Safety factors: Turning the hands inward or outward increases stress to the wrists and elbows. If neutral spinal alignment is difficult to maintain, modify the exercise. The most common error is the loss of core stabilization.

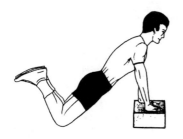 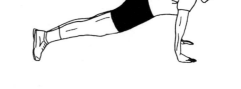

Fig. 10.8–Knee push-up   *Fig. 10.9–Full body push-up*

Modifications (easiest to hardest): wall push-up, hands and knees (table-top) push-up, knee push-up with hands on weightroom bench, knee push-up with hands on aerobic step, knee push-up with hands on floor, knee push-up with knees elevated (decline), full body push-up with hands on bench, full body push-up with hands on floor, full body push-up with feet elevated (decline), full body decline push-up with weights on back

Note: In any position, the closer the hands are together, the greater the triceps involvement.

Chest Exercise Machines

Chest press: flat, incline or seated

- Muscles worked, joint actions, etc. are the same as those for bench press.

- When adjusting machine, be sure the bar handles are aligned with or slightly above nipples.

- Alignment and technique, joints stabilized, etc. are the same as those for bench press. Exhale on the way up (or out).

Pec dec: flat, incline or seated

- Muscles worked, joint actions, etc. are the same as those for the dumbbell fly.

- Adjust machine so that the upper arms are perpendicular to the torso. Keep wrists, forearms and elbows in contact with the pads; use forearms when pushing.

- Keep in mind that this exercise is high risk for clients with shoulder problems since most machines take the shoulder joint to an extreme range of external rotation and horizontal extension. This places the shoulder in a vulnerable position. Have clients move slowly through the eccentric phase and assist them when entering and leaving the machine if necessary. Avoid spinal or hip flexion; keep head, shoulders and buttocks pressed against the pad.

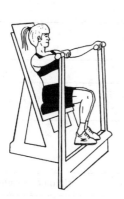
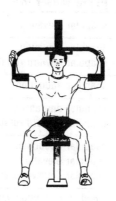
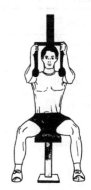

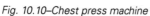

Fig. 10.10–Chest press machine   *Fig. 10.11–Pec dec machine*

▼ Exercises for the Upper Back ▼

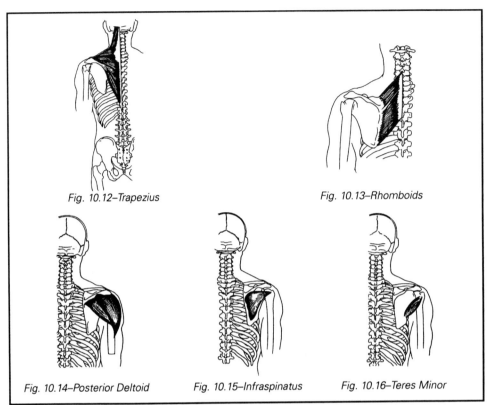

Fig. 10.12–Trapezius

Fig. 10.13–Rhomboids

Fig. 10.14–Posterior Deltoid

Fig. 10.15–Infraspinatus

Fig. 10.16–Teres Minor

Muscle	Prime Mover for:	Assists with:
Trapezius I	scapular elevation	
Trapezius II	scapular elevation scapular upward rotation	
Trapezius III	scapular adduction	
Trapezius IV	scapular depression scapular upward rotation	
Rhomboids	scapular adduction scapular elevation scapular downward rotation	
Posterior Deltoid	shoulder horizontal extension	shoulder extension
Teres Minor and Infraspinatus	shoulder horizontal extension shoulder external rotation	

The following upper back exercises are important to work from a functional perspective. Common weightroom exercises for the pectoralis major (e.g., bench press, flys, push-ups) may result in postural misalignment if performed excessively without working the opposing muscle groups. Specifically, tight anterior muscles may cause excessive scapular abduction (protraction) and shoulder internal rotation (the powerful latissimus dorsi is also an internal rotator of the shoulder joint). In addition, kyphosis (rounded, hunched back) is a common postural misalignment among non-exercisers, and the following exercises are useful as a corrective.

Reverse Fly

Equipment used: dumbbells, flat or incline bench

Moving joints	Joint action	Muscles worked
shoulders	horizontal extension	posterior deltoid, infraspinatus, teres minor
scapulae	adduction (retraction)	trapezius III, rhomboids

1. Starting position: Lie prone on flat or incline bench, or seated on bench (bend over, flexing at hips). Keep neck and spine in neutral alignment. Support back either on bench (prone), or on thighs (seated). Start with arms down, palms facing each other.

2. Moving joints: Shoulders and scapulae move. Stabilize spine (no spinal rotation with extension) and neck. Avoid looking up and hyperextending neck. Elbows are stabilized in a slightly flexed position.

3. Alignment and technique: Keep upper arm perpendicular to torso, lead with elbows and move up slightly beyond the shoulder joint range of motion and into conscious scapular adduction. Another variation is to start with scapular adduction, and then perform the shoulder joint movement (horizontal extension). Stay in the horizontal plane. Exhale on the upward movement and control the descent.

4. Engage and contract the posterior deltoid, and especially the mid-trapezius and rhomboids.

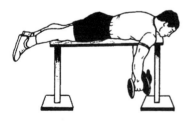 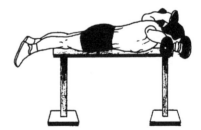

Fig. 10.17–Prone reverse fly on flat bench

5.   Safety factors: Keep movement slow and controlled to avoid shoulder injury. Watch for tendency to adduct and extend the shoulder joint in the sagittal plane, especially if weights are too heavy (this allows the latissimus dorsi to help out). Most clients will need to start this exercise with little or no weight. Watch for neck hyperextension and wrist breaking. Avoid the seated, hip flexed position if clients are unable to adequately support the torso either with the abdominals and erector spinae, or on thighs.

Spotting guidelines: If client is seated, spot from behind. If client is prone, kneel in front of bench. Spot forearms or wrists. Remind client to lead with elbows. Palpating the scapular adductors and posterior deltoids may help clients stay focused.

Horizontal Seated Row

Equipment used: low pulley machine, horizontal seated row machine, or tubing

Moving joints	Joint action	Muscles worked
shoulders	horizontal extension	posterior deltoid, infraspinatus, teres minor
scapulae	adduction (retraction)	trapezius III, rhomboids
elbows	flexion	biceps, brachialis, brachioradialis

1. Starting position: Sit with hip flexed at 90°, spine in neutral alignment. If seated on floor, flex knees slightly to assist with good seated posture. Use grips or a bar that allows palms to pronate and face down. Start with elbows extended and arms in horizontal plane.

2. Moving joints: Shoulders, scapulae, and elbows. Keep entire spine in neutral, avoid extending spine or hips. Wrists are neutral.

3. Alignment and technique: When rowing, lead backwards with elbows. Keep upper arm in horizontal plane and consciously go back into scapular movement (or scapular movement can precede the arm/shoulder movement). Exhale when pulling back, and control the eccentric phase.

4. Engage and contract the posterior deltoids and consciously contract the mid-trapezius muscles and rhomboids.

5. Safety factors and common errors: Many people confuse this exercise with seated latissimus dorsi rows. To target the posterior deltoids, trapezius muscles, and rhomboids, stay in the horizontal plane—elbows lifted. Watch for wrist breaking (pulling with the wrists), and rocking with the lower spine. Avoid fly-away weight stacks.

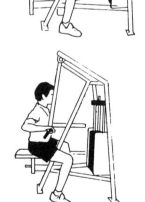

Spotting guidelines: Spot from behind, holding forearms if necessary. As the client brings his/her elbows back, guide elbows into horizontal plane. Palpating the scapular adductors may be helpful.

Fig. 10.18–Seated horizontal row

Bent Elbow Reverse Fly Machine

Equipment used: reverse fly/row machine

Moving joints	Joint action	Muscles worked
shoulders	horizontal extension	posterior deltoid infraspinatus, teres minor
scapulae	adduction (retraction)	trapezius III, rhomboids

1. Starting position: Sit with hips flexed at 90°, spine in neutral, and abdominals contracted. Adjust seat so that upper arms are perpendicular to torso and movement occurs in the horizontal plane. Forearms are crossed; palms face floor.

2. Moving joints: Shoulders and scapulae move. Neck, spine and elbows are stabilized. Keep scapulae depressed.

3. Alignment and technique: Exhale on backward movement, taking scapulae through full range of adduction. Inhale and control the forward movement (eccentric phase).

4. Engage and contract the scapular adductors, as well as the posterior deltoids, through both concentric and eccentric phases.

5. Safety factors: Make certain torso is in contact with pad and the neck and upper trapezius muscles are relaxed.

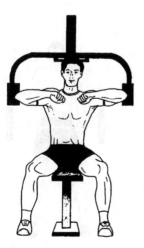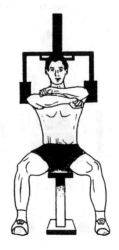

Fig. 10.19–Machine reverse fly exercise

Shoulder Shrugs

Equipment used: dumbbells, barbell or machine (may use a Universal-type bench press station)

Moving joints	Joint action	Muscles worked
scapulae (shoulder girdle)	elevation	trapezius I and II, rhomboids, and levator scapulae

1. Starting position: Sit or stand with feet shoulder-width apart for stability. If using barbell, place hands directly in line with shoulders (some trainers recommend holding the barbell behind the body for the optimal line of pull). If standing, knees are slightly flexed, with neck, spine and pelvis in neutral, abdominals in.

2. Moving joints: Shoulder girdle. All other joints are stabilized. Elbows and wrists have no independent movement.

3. Alignment and technique: Start with shoulder girdle depressed, elevate it in straight line up towards ears. Many strength training experts recommend inhaling when elevating shoulders and exhaling on the descent.

4. Engage and contract the upper trapezius muscles, levator scapulae, and rhomboids.

5. Safety factors: Avoid swinging the weights or assisting the lift with torso or leg movement. Watch for head ducking (forward head) or jerking the head backwards.

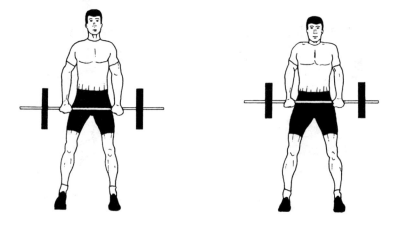

Fig. 10.20–Shoulder shrugs with barbell

▼ Exercises for the Shoulders ▼

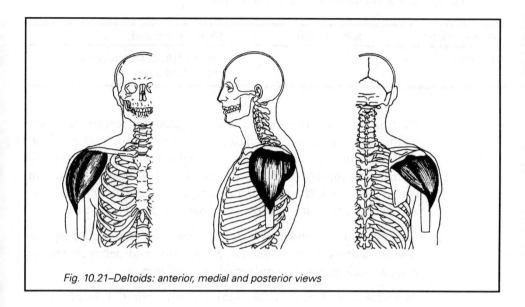

Fig. 10.21–Deltoids: anterior, medial and posterior views

Muscle	Prime Mover for:	Assists with:
Anterior Deltoid	shoulder flexion shoulder horizontal flexion	shoulder internal rotation
Medial Deltoid	shoulder abduction shoulder horizontal extension	
Posterior Deltoid	shoulder horizontal extension	shoulder extension shoulder external rotation

Front Raises

Equipment used: dumbbells or barbell, bench

Moving joints	Joint action	Muscles worked
shoulders	flexion	anterior deltoid, pectoralis major (clavicular portion)

1. Starting position: Stand or sit. In standing position, feet are shoulder-width apart, knees slightly flexed, with neck, spine and pelvis in neutral alignment. Elbows are fully extended but not hyperextended; palms are pronated with dumbbells or barbell against thighs. In seated position, feet are flat on floor, hips are flexed at 90°, and spine and neck are in neutral. Scapulae are depressed and adducted.

2. Moving joints: Shoulders. Wrists and elbows are stabilized. Scapulae remain depressed and adducted. Neck, spine and pelvis remain in neutral; abdominals are contracted to stabilize spine.

3. Alignment and technique: May be performed bilaterally or unilaterally. Palms remain pronated throughout movement. Flex shoulders until arms are above shoulder height (some experts recommend flexing until arms are overhead). Exhale during the upward movement.

4. Engage and contract the anterior deltoids and the upper pectorals throughout both the concentric and eccentric phases.

5. Safety factors: Seated, unilateral front raises are safer for the back than standing, bilateral raises. If client is standing, take care to ensure that the torso is stable and that there is no momentum. Watch that the neck maintains a neutral position. Avoid wrist breaking.

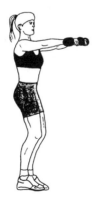

    Spotting guidelines: Stand in front of client, spotting the weights. Remind client to depress and adduct scapulae.

Fig. 10.22–Standing front raises

Lateral Raises

Equipment used: dumbbells, bench

Moving joints	Joint action	Muscles worked
shoulders	abduction	medial deltoid, supraspinatus
scapulae	upward rotation	trapezius II and IV, serratus anterior

1. Starting position: Stand or sit. In standing position, feet are shoulder width apart, knees slightly flexed, with neck, spine and pelvis in neutral alignment. In seated position, feet are flat on floor, hips are flexed at 90°, and neck and spine are in neutral. In both positions, scapulae are adducted and depressed; elbows are slightly flexed, and wrists are neutral (arms hang down at sides, palms facing thighs).

2. Moving joints: Shoulders. Wrists and elbows are stabilized. Scapulae remain depressed and adducted, neck stays in neutral. There should be no movement of the spine or legs.

3. Alignment and technique: As the shoulders are abducted, maintain partial shoulder external rotation (palms should face the floor), and abduct shoulders only to 90° (the greater the abduction, the more important the external rotation). Lead with the elbows, not the wrists. Exhale on the way up (concentric phase).

4. Engage and contract the deltoids throughout both the concentric and the eccentric phases.

5. Safety factors: Abducting the shoulders beyond 90° while maintaining internal rotation may lead to impingement syndrome (the greater tubercle of the humerus abuts the acromion process and irritates soft tissue structures, especially the supraspinatus tendon). Watch for errors, such as initiating the movement with the legs or torso, ducking the head forward during abduction, unstable scapulae, and wrist breaking.

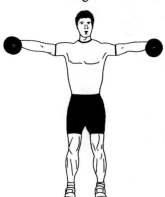

Fig. 10.23–Standing lateral raise

Spotting guidelines: Stand behind client and spot the forearms, wrists, or weights. Remind client to lead with the elbows, not the wrists.

Overhead Press (Military or Standing Press)

Equipment used: dumbbells or barbell, bench

Moving joints	Joint action	Muscles worked
shoulders	abduction	deltoids, supraspinatus
scapulae	upward rotation	trapezius II and IV, serratus anterior
elbows	extension	triceps

1. Starting position: Sit or stand. In the seated position, feet must be flat on floor, hips flexed at 90°, spine neutral, scapulae depressed and adducted. Starting position is down, with shoulders externally rotated and palms pronated (if using dumbbells, palms also may be mid-pronated, facing ears); hands are slightly wider than shoulder-width apart.

2. Moving joints: Shoulders, scapulae and elbows. Spine and neck should be stabilized. If standing, knees should be slightly flexed, pelvis neutral, and the lower body should be stabilized. Wrists stay in neutral, and shoulder elevation is minimized.

3. Alignment and technique: Exhale when pressing up. Fully extend elbows without hyperextending them. May be performed bilaterally or unilaterally. Try to lift weights up over the top of the head while maintaining scapular adduction and depression. With a barbell, lightly touch the clavicle and press up in front of the face.

4. Engage and contract the deltoids and triceps. Isometrically contract the scapular adductors, as well as the pectoralis minor and trapezius IV to maintain depression.

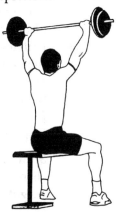

Fig. 10.24–Seated military press with barbell

5. Safety factors: The behind-the-neck military press has become controversial due to the vulnerable position of the shoulder joint (horizontally extended and externally rotated behind the frontal plane). To reduce the risk of injury, perform the exercise in front of the head. Avoid wrist breaking and leaning backward (a posterior lean is common with heavy weights). Watch for excessive shoulder girdle elevation and abduction; keep the head and neck in neutral alignment.

Spotting guidelines: With dumbbells, stand or sit behind client and cup the elbows or spot the forearms. With barbell, stand behind and track the barbell with hands.

Upright Row

Equipment used: dumbbells or barbell

Moving joints	Joint action	Muscles worked
shoulders	abduction	deltoids, supraspinatus
scapulae	upward rotation	trapezius II and IV, serratus anterior
elbows	flexion	biceps
Optional: scapulae	elevation	trapezius I and II, rhomboids and levator scapulae

1. Starting position: Stand with feet shoulder-width apart, knees slightly flexed, pelvis, spine, and neck in neutral position, and abdominals contracted. Hands are in a pronated, narrow grip (no more than four inches apart) in front of thighs. Starting position is down.

2. Moving joints: Shoulders, scapulae and elbows move. Elevation of the scapulae at the beginning or at the end of the range of motion is an option if upper trapezius strengthening is a goal (otherwise, keep scapulae depressed). Wrists stay as neutral as possible. Stabilize lower body, keep abdominals contracted.

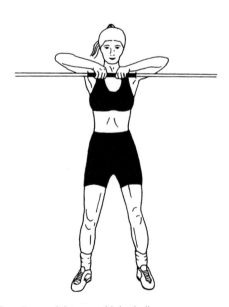

Fig. 10.25–Standing upright row with barbell

3. Alignment and technique: Lead with elbows, not wrists. Keep barbell or dumbbells close to the body. If upper trapezius work is a goal, lift elbows above shoulder level and elevate scapulae; otherwise, shoulder abduction occurs to only about 90°. Exhale when lifting up.

4. Engage and contract the deltoids, biceps and possibly the upper trapezius muscles.

5. Safety factors: A typical problem with this exercise is the tendency to lead with the wrists and keep elbows down, placing great stress on the wrists. Watch shoulder abduction above 90° in clients with shoulder problems. Avoid leaning backwards.

Spotting guidelines: Stand behind client, hands tracking close to bar in a wide grip. Remind client to lead with elbows.

Shoulder Exercise Machines

Overhead Press

■ The exerciser is usually in seated position. Machine may be part of a multi-unit setup, or may be a variable resistance single station type machine.

■ Muscles worked, moving joints, joints stabilized, alignment, etc. are the same as those for the free weight overhead press.

■ Adjust seat height so that handles are level with shoulder joint.

■ If machine has a back pad, press hips, shoulders and head against the pad and maintain contracted abdominals. If there is no back pad, take care to keep the torso and neck in neutral alignment, and avoid leaning backwards.

■ Multi-unit shoulder presses may be used facing either toward or away from the weight stack. Depending on where the stool is placed, facing away may be riskier for the shoulder joint (if shoulders are horizontally extended and externally rotated behind the frontal plane).

■ Avoid hyperextending or snapping the elbows during extension.

Lateral Raise

■ The exerciser is in the seated position.

■ Muscles worked, moving joints, joints stabilized, alignment, etc. are the same as those for free weight lateral raises.

■ Adjust seat height so that the cam or pivot point is aligned with the shoulder joint.

■ Press hips, shoulders and head back against pad.

■ Maintain pressure against arm pads with the lateral aspect of the arms and lead with the elbows. Avoid lifting with the wrists.

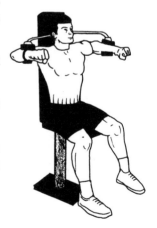

Fig. 10.26–Seated lateral raise

▼ Exercises for the Rotator Cuff Muscles ▼

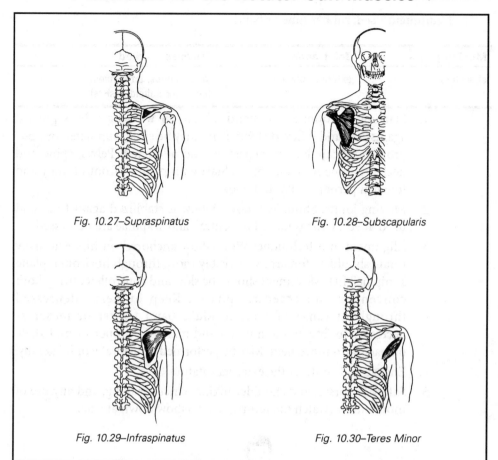

Fig. 10.27–Supraspinatus

Fig. 10.28–Subscapularis

Fig. 10.29–Infraspinatus

Fig. 10.30–Teres Minor

Muscle	Prime Mover for:	Assists with:
Supraspinatus	shoulder abduction	
Subscapularis	shoulder internal rotation	
Infraspinatus	shoulder external rotation shoulder horizontal extension	
Teres Minor	shoulder external rotation shoulder horizontal extension	

External Rotation with Tube

Equipment used: rubber tube or band

Moving joints	Joint action	Muscles worked
shoulders	external rotation	infraspinatus, teres minor (posterior deltoid assists)

1. Starting position: Sit or stand. Elbow on working side is pressed against hip and is flexed at 90°. Palm may be either supinated or mid-pronated. Scapulae are depressed and adducted. Pelvis, spine and neck are in neutral alignment. Start with palm in front of body and forearm perpendicular to torso.

2. Moving joints: Shoulders move. Elbow is stabilized against hip and fixed at 90°, wrist is locked in neutral, and scapulae are depressed.

3. Alignment and technique: With elbow anchored on hip, externally rotate shoulder (forearm will visibly move through horizontal plane at hip height). Movement should be slow and controlled during both concentric and eccentric phases. Keep humerus depressed throughout range of motion. Make band tighter or looser as necessary to fatigue the muscles and maintain proper form. Exhale on backward movement. May be performed unilaterally or bilaterally.

4. Engage and contract the external rotators.

5. Safety factors: Avoid shoulder hiking, wrist breaking, and any use of momentum (watch the return). Keep elbow down at side.

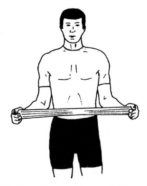

Fig. 10.31–Standing external rotation with tubing

Note: It is probably not as important to perform isolation type exercises for the internal rotator cuff muscles. These muscles (subscapularis and teres major) are assisted by many other powerful muscles, including: anterior deltoid, pectoralis major, biceps and the latissimus dorsi.

▼ Exercises for the Middle Back ▼

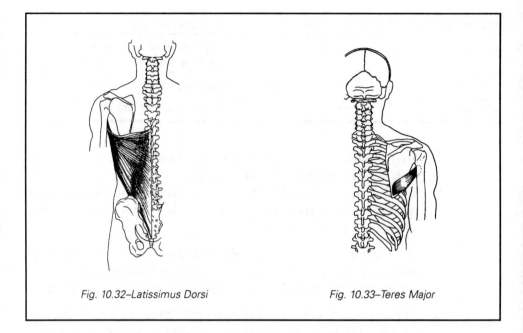

Fig. 10.32–Latissimus Dorsi   *Fig. 10.33–Teres Major*

Muscle	Prime Mover for:	Assists with:
Latissimus Dorsi	shoulder extension shoulder adduction	shoulder internal rotation shoulder horizontal extension
Teres Major	shoulder extension shoulder adduction shoulder internal rotation	shoulder horizontal extension

Lat Pull-down (wide grip)

Equipment used: high pulley or lat pull-down machine

Moving joints	Joint action	Muscles worked
shoulders	adduction	latissimus dorsi, teres major, sternal portion of pectoralis major
scapulae	downward rotation	pectoralis minor, rhomboids
elbows	flexion	biceps, brachialis, brachioradialis

1. Starting position: Sit or kneel. If seated, knees are placed under knee pad, hips are flexed at 90°, and spine and neck are in neutral. If kneeling, pelvis should be held in neutral position (avoid hip or spinal flexion). Start in up position, hands in wide, pronated grip, scapulae adducted and depressed.

2. Moving joints: Shoulders, scapulae and elbows. Stabilize scapulae so as to avoid elevation and abduction. Keep head and neck in a natural extension of the spine; keep spine stabilized and wrists in neutral.

3. Alignment and technique: Exhale on pull-down. In the behind-the-neck lat pull-down, bar should touch base of neck (neck must stay in neutral). When pulling bar to the front, pull toward the sternum. Elbows should stay away from the body during pull-down. Release bar upwards slowly, with control, keeping the scapulae depressed.

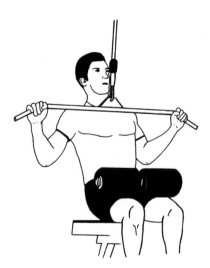

Fig. 10.34–Seated lat pull-down

4. Engage and contract the latissimus dorsi prior to the pull-down, maintaining a conscious contraction on the way down and on the way up.

5. Safety factors: Use care when training a client with the behind-the-neck lat pull-down; this exercise places the shoulder joint in the vulnerable position of horizontal extension and external rotation behind the frontal plane and is therefore on the "high risk" list for many sports medicine practitioners. In addition, many clients don't have adequate shoulder flexibility to stay in good alignment; they hunch over and duck their neck during back lat pull-downs. Using the pull-down in front may be preferable. However, watch the tendency to lean backward and rock the pelvis. Avoid wrist breaking.

Spotting guidelines: Stand behind client with hands pronated above the bar. Encourage client to depress scapulae throughout.

Bent Over Row (unilateral)

Equipment used: dumbbell, bench

Moving joints	Joint action	Muscles worked
shoulder	extension	latissimus dorsi, teres major, sternal portion of pectoralis major (posterior deltoid and long head of triceps assist)
elbow	flexion	biceps, brachialis, brachioradialis

Note: Trapezius III and rhomboids contract strongly isometrically as stabilizers due to anti-gravity position.

1. Starting position: Half-kneel on bench. Same side hand and knee are on bench; working side has extended leg with foot on floor. Dumbbell is held with mid-pronated palm (facing bench). Prior to movement, adduct and depress scapulae. Spine should be in neutral and parallel to floor, with head and neck in a natural extension of the spine.

2. Moving joints: Shoulder and elbow. Unless the goal is to work the mid-trapezius muscles and rhomboids, the scapulae should remain stabilized. Spine and neck are stabilized, abdominals are contracted.

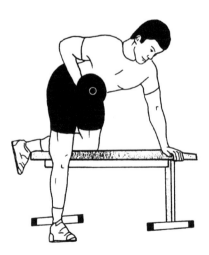

Fig. 10.35–Bent over row (knee on bench)

3. Alignment and technique: Exhale as the weight is lifted; keep the working arm close to the body. Lower the weight slowly, with control, maintaining scapular adduction.

4. Engage and contract the latissimus dorsi and the biceps. Consciously contract the mid-trapezius and rhomboids isometrically throughout exercise.

5. Safety factors: Many clients tend to drop the weight too quickly, lose scapular stabilization, and "peck" at the weight (duck their head). Avoid spinal rotation and extension as the weight is lifted. Keep wrists in neutral and avoid locking the elbow during extension. Watch the tendency to hunch the shoulders.

Spotting guidelines: Stand or kneel at client's side, spot forearm or weight. Remind client to keep scapulae adducted.

Seated Lat Row (Low Row)

Equipment used: low pulley or seated row machine

Moving joints	Joint action	Muscles worked
shoulders	extension	latissimus dorsi, teres major, sternal portion of pectoralis major (posterior deltoid and long head of triceps assist)
elbows	flexion	biceps, brachialis, brachioradialis
Optional: scapulae	adduction	trapezius III, rhomboids

1. Starting position: Sit with hips flexed at 90°, spine and neck in neutral. If seated on floor or low pad, knees should be flexed. Start with arms out in shoulder flexion, elbows soft, and palms in mid-pronation (facing each other, thumbs up). If using a bar, take a narrow, pronated grip. Depress and adduct scapulae.

2. Moving joints: Shoulders and elbows. Scapulae can either be stabilized (mid-trapezius muscles and rhomboids contract isometrically), or can actively abduct and adduct, depending on goals. Keep shoulder girdle depressed. Hold the lower back still and stabilize the torso and neck for optimal latissimus dorsi isolation.

3. Alignment and technique: Exhale when pulling back; pull handles to lower chest. Make sure torso remains upright through both concentric and eccentric phases.

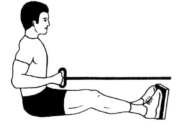 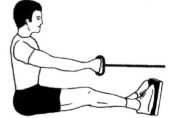

Fig. 10.36–Low pulley seated lat row

4. Engage and contract the latissimus dorsi and biceps. Focus on either contracting the scapular adductors isometrically (to help isolate the latissimus dorsi), or isotonically through full range (if goal is to work the trapezius muscles).

5. Safety factors: Many clients tend to perform "low back" rows. This is not appropriate if the goal is to work the latissimus dorsi and/or trapezius muscles. Locked knees in the low sit position increases stress to the low back. Avoid fly-away weights, especially on the return.

Spotting guidelines: Kneel behind client and spot forearms.

Lat Pull-over

Equipment used: barbell or dumbbell, bench

Moving joints	Joint action	Muscles worked
shoulders	extension	latissimus dorsi, teres major, sternal portion of pectoralis major (posterior deltoid and long head of triceps assist)
scapulae	depression downward rotation upward tilt	pectoralis minor, trapezius IV pectoralis minor, rhomboids pectoralis minor

1. Starting position: Lie supine on bench, feet flat on floor or on bench. The end of the bench should just support the base of the skull; neck should maintain natural alignment. Abdominals are contracted to maintain neutral spine throughout exercise. Hold barbell with narrow, pronated grip over the lower chest; elbows are flexed at sides, wrists locked. If holding dumbbell, cup end of dumbbell with both hands, hold over lower chest.

2. Moving joints: Shoulders and scapulae. Stabilize spine, neck and pelvis. Stabilize elbows in flexed position.

3. Alignment and technique: Stay in sagittal plane and move weight over face, behind head, and toward the floor. Exhale as elbows are pulled back toward sides of chest. Keep movement slow and controlled.

4. Engage and contract the latissimus dorsi and lower pectorals. Keep abdominals isometrically contracted throughout exercise.

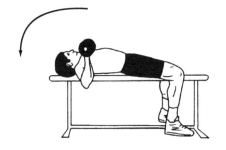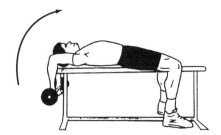

Fig. 10.37–Lat pull-over with barbell

5. Safety factors: Be very cautious with heavy weights; proper spotting is essential to prevent shoulder injury. Perform the exercise slowly and use great control during the eccentric phase. Also, since the weight passes over the client's face, care is required. Avoid arching the lower back; contract abdominals. Keep arms in sagittal plane; avoid flaring the elbows out.

Spotting guidelines: Kneel or stand behind client's head, tracking barbell with hands. Encourage client to maintain abdominal tightness.

▼ Exercises for the Arms ▼

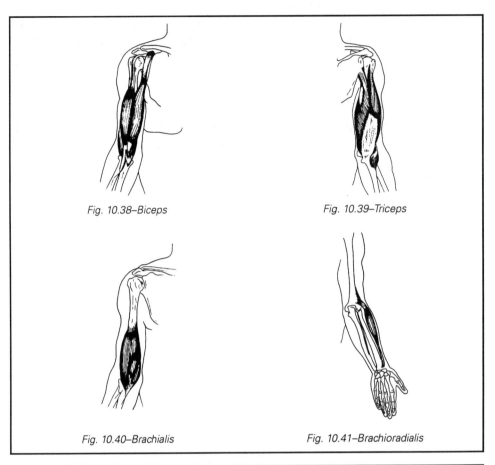

Fig. 10.38–Biceps

Fig. 10.39–Triceps

Fig. 10.40–Brachialis

Fig. 10.41–Brachioradialis

Muscle	Prime Mover for:	Assists with:
Biceps Brachii	elbow flexion	radio-ulnar supination shoulder flexion shoulder internal rotation shoulder horizontal flexion shoulder abduction shoulder adduction
Brachialis	elbow flexion	
Brachioradialis	elbow flexion	
Triceps Brachii	elbow extension	shoulder extension shoulder adduction

Triceps Kickback (unilateral)

Equipment used: dumbbell, bench

Moving joints	Joint action	Muscles worked
elbow	extension	triceps

Note: Latissimus dorsi, teres major, mid-trapezius muscles, and rhomboids all contract strongly isometrically due to anti-gravity position.

1. Starting position: Half kneel on bench. Same side hand and knee are on bench; working side has extended leg with foot flat on floor. Dumbbell is held with mid-pronated palm, facing bench. Scapulae are depressed and adducted, shoulder joint is extended so that upper arm is parallel to floor. Elbow is flexed at 90° with wrist straight.

2. Moving joints: Elbow moves while shoulder joint and shoulder girdle are stabilized. Wrist is stabilized in neutral (straight) position. Abdominals are contracted so that the spine maintains neutral alignment and the head and neck maintain a natural extension of the spine.

3. Alignment and technique: Exhale as the elbow extends. Elbow should extend fully, without hyperextension. Movement should be slow and controlled. Optional radio-ulnar joint movement to full pronation may provide more gravitational resistance for long head of the triceps.

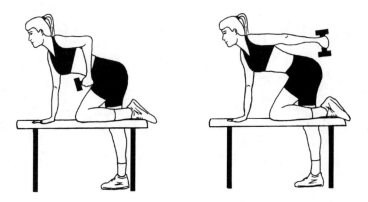

Fig. 10.42–Unilateral triceps kickback on bench

4. Engage and contract the triceps. Isometrically contract the latissimus dorsi, teres major, posterior deltoid, mid-trapezius and rhomboids.

5. Safety factors: Avoid wrist flexing and extending. Even with optional pronation, wrist should remain neutral. Avoid hunching shoulder, hyperextending neck, and spinal rotation with extension. Watch for "slamming" elbow joint into full extension; movement should always be smooth and controlled.

Spotting guidelines: Spot client from working side; assist forearm or weight.

Standing Triceps Press-down

Equipment used: high pulley

Moving joints	Joint action	Muscles worked
elbows	extension	triceps

1. Starting position: Stand with knees slightly flexed and with pelvis, spine and neck in neutral alignment. Bring lat bar or ropes down to shoulder level; elbows are flexed and touch sides of ribs. Hands are approximately six inches apart and pronated.

2. Moving joints: Elbows. Torso is stabilized with abdominals contracted. Elbows remain pressed into sides of body. Shoulders are stabilized so that neither flexion nor abduction is possible. Scapulae are depressed throughout exercise. Wrists are neutral.

3. Alignment and technique: Exhale as elbows extend and bar is pressed down. Elbows should fully extend without hyper- extending. Slowly return to start, flexing elbows and maintaining contact with sides of body.

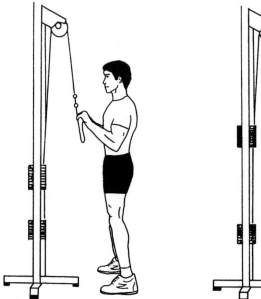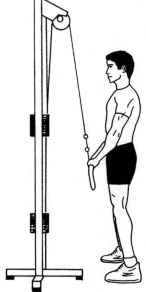

Fig. 10.43–Standing triceps press-down

4. Engage and contract the triceps. Isometrically contract the lower trapezius muscles and the pectoralis minor to maintain scapular depression; and keep the latissimus dorsi contracted to maintain a neutral shoulder position.

5. Safety factors: Avoid fly-away weights, especially during the eccentric phase. Watch that the torso does not rock back and forth. One of the most common errors is allowing the shoulders to flex and abduct as the bar is raised. Avoid scapular elevation and wrist breaking.

Spotting guidelines: Stand behind client, ready to assist with pronated, wide grip. Remind client to depress scapulae and to use only triceps.

Standing Triceps Extension (French Press)

Equipment used: barbell or dumbbell

Moving joints	Joint action	Muscles worked
elbows	extension	triceps

1. Starting position: Sit or stand. If standing, knees must be flexed and abdominals contracted, with pelvis, spine and neck in neutral. Hold barbell with pronated, close grip (hands no more than six inches apart). If using dumbbell, cup one end of the dumbbell with both hands. Start with weight overhead and elbows extended; elbows are held close to ears. Wrists are neutral. Scapulae are depressed.

2. Moving joints: Elbows. All other joints are stabilized, including: shoulders, wrists, neck, spine and pelvis.

3. Alignment and technique: Flexing the elbows, slowly lower the barbell behind the head to the tops of shoulders. Maintain the upper arm position: elbows point straight to ceiling and are pressed in (to sides of head). Exhale as elbows extend. May be performed bilaterally or unilaterally.

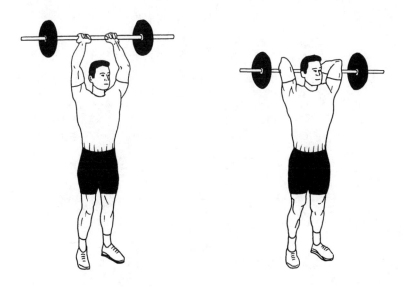

Fig. 10.44–Standing bilateral French press with barbell

4. Engage and contract the triceps throughout both concentric and eccentric phases. Maintain lower trapezius and pectoralis minor isometric tension, as well as tight abdominals.

5. Safety factors: Avoid lower body movement such as pushing with the knees or flexing the spine. Shoulder flexibility is required to place the upper arm in the proper position. Clients who are unable to stay in correct alignment should be given another exercise. Due to lack of flexibility, scapulae may elevate, shoulders may not fully flex, and it may be difficult to keep elbows close to head. Avoid ducking the head and wrist breaking.

Spotting guidelines: Stand behind client, tracking bar with alternate grip.

Supine Elbow Extension

Equipment used: barbell or dumbbells, bench

Moving joints	Joint action	Muscles worked
elbows	extension	triceps

1. Starting position: Lie supine on bench with feet flat on floor or up on bench. Abdominals are contracted to help maintain neutral spinal alignment. Barbell is held with pronated, close grip (hands no more than six inches apart), and shoulders are flexed at 90° with forearms, wrists and hands in straight line. Single dumbbell is cupped on one end with both hands. If using two dumbbells, start in pronation.

2. Moving joints: Elbows move. Shoulders and upper arms are held stable, wrists are neutral and spine is stabilized on bench.

3. Alignment and technique: Keeping elbows pointed toward ceiling, slowly lower the weight to forehead or top of head (dumbbell is lowered just behind head). Exhale as elbows extend. If using two dumbbells, lower weight into mid-pronated grip so that palms face ears. Extend and return to full pronation.

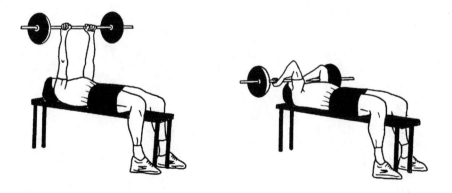

Fig. 10.45–Supine elbow extension with barbell

4. Engage and contract the triceps. Maintain a secure abdominal contraction (isometric) throughout the exercise.

5. Safety factors: Avoid the tendency to extend the shoulders and use the latissimus dorsi. Keep the upper arms completely stationary; do not let elbows flare out. Avoid wrist breaking. Emphasize control during the eccentric phase to prevent potential head injuries.

Spotting guidelines: Stand behind client's head, with knees flexed. Be prepared to kneel during client's eccentric phase as you spot the weight. Use an alternate grip on the barbell.

Triceps Dip

Equipment used: dip bars or bench

Moving joints	Joint action	Muscles worked
elbows	extension	triceps
shoulders	flexion	anterior deltoid, pectoralis major

Note: Trapezius IV and pectoralis minor contract isometrically quite strongly to keep shoulder girdle from elevating

1. Starting position: Hands are placed on bars (or bench) with elbows straight but not hyperextended. Scapulae are depressed and adducted. Abdominals are contracted and body hangs in neutral with knees bent (ankles may be crossed). If using bench, hands should be on edge of bench, with hips close in front. Knees may be bent or straight.

2. Moving joints: Elbows and shoulders. All other joints should be stabilized, with special focus on scapular stabilization. If using bench, stabilize lower body so that the work is performed by the triceps and shoulder flexors.

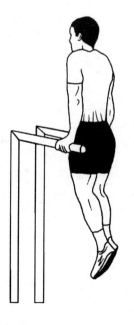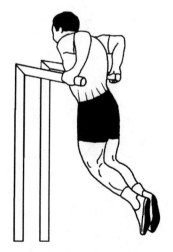

Fig. 10.46–Triceps dip on dip bars

3. Alignment and technique: Lower the body until the elbows are flexed at 90° and the upper arms are parallel to the floor. Exhale as elbows extend and lift body. Keep the elbow and shoulder movement in the sagittal plane; do not let the elbows flare out.

4. Engage and contract the triceps, anterior deltoids, and pectorals. Engage the lower trapezius muscles and the pectoralis minor to keep scapulae depressed.

5. Safety factors: Avoid overbending (hyperflexing) or hyperextending the elbow joint in a weight bearing position as this causes joint stress. Watch for tendency to hunch (elevate) the shoulders; keep elbows close to sides. If using a bench, do not allow the client to "cheat" by lifting and lowering with his/her legs. Let the lower body hang so that all the weight is lifted by the appropriate muscles.

Alternate Dumbbell Biceps Curl

Equipment used: dumbbells

Moving joints	Joint action	Muscles worked
elbows	flexion	biceps, brachialis, brachioradialis
radio-ulnar	supination	supinator

1. Starting position: Stand or sit. In standing position, the knees are slightly flexed, with pelvis, spine and neck in neutral. If seated, hips are flexed 90°, with spine and neck in neutral. Shoulder girdle is depressed and adducted. Palms face sides of body (mid-pronation).

2. Moving joints: elbows and radio-ulnar joints. Shoulders do not move; scapulae, neck, spine, etc. are stabilized. Wrists stay neutral.

3. Alignment and technique: Exhale as one elbow slowly flexes. Palm supinates gradually as weight is lifted. Gradually return back to mid-pronation as weight is lowered. Repeat with other side.

4. Engage and contract the biceps. Maintain the contraction throughout both concentric and eccentric phases.

5. Safety factors and common errors: Avoid wrist breaking (no flexing or extending); this may lead to tennis elbow and/or carpal tunnel syndrome. Keep upper arm still. Many clients "cheat" by throwing the arms forward or by pulling the elbows backward (in this case, have them lift a lighter weight). Watch tendency to arch low back and/or lock knees while curling. Keep shoulders down. Be aware that slowly alternating heavy weights in this exercise creates increasing tension in forearm muscles, which isometrically contract to maintain grip on dumbbells.

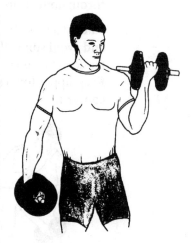

Spotting guidelines: Stand behind client, spotting forearms if necessary. Touch backs of elbows as a reminder to stabilize.

Fig. 10.47–Standing alternate dumbbell biceps curl

Concentration Curl

Equipment used: dumbbell, bench

Moving joints	Joint action	Muscles worked
elbows	flexion	biceps, brachialis, brachioradialis

1. Starting position: Sit, placing elbow of working arm on inside of thigh. Opposite hand is placed either on opposite thigh or behind working arm for support. Feet are flat on floor and hips are flexed. Spine and neck are in neutral with scapulae depressed. Dumbbell is held with a supinated grip and neutral wrist. Start with elbow extended.

2. Moving joints: Elbows. Wrist is kept straight, shoulder is stabilized. Spine and neck are stabilized.

3. Alignment and technique: Hinge from hips, not waist, so that spine is in neutral alignment (slightly anteriorly tilt the pelvis). Exhale as elbow flexes; bring weight up to shoulder. Slowly lower, inhaling. This exercise may place slightly more emphasis on the short head of the biceps due to the internally rotated position of the shoulder (the short head assists with internal shoulder rotation).

4. Engage and contract the biceps, brachialis, and the brachioradialis throughout entire exercise.

5. Safety factors: Avoid using torso movement to perform the exercise, and avoid spinal flexion and hunching over. Some clients may have a tendency to push the shoulder joint forward (abduct the scapula). Keep upper torso still. As with all biceps exercises, wrist breaking is a concern.

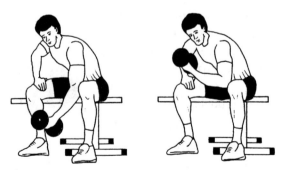

Fig. 10.48–Seated concentration curl

Preacher Bench Curls

Equipment used: preacher curl bench with barbell (may use EZ curl bar) or dumbbells

Moving joints	Joint action	Muscles worked
elbows	flexion	biceps, brachialis, brachioradialis

1. Starting position: Sit facing preacher bench. Bench should be adjusted so that shoulders are flexed about 45°. Upper arms rest on pad. Sit so that hips are flexed into slight anterior pelvic tilt and rib cage rests on pad. Grip barbell or dumbbells with supinated palms. Press shoulders down. Start with elbows extended.

2. Moving joints: Elbows. Stabilize shoulder girdle, neck and spine. Keep wrists in neutral.

3. Alignment and technique: Exhale as elbows flex through as full a range of motion as possible. Slowly lower, inhaling.

4. Engage and contract the biceps, brachialis, and brachioradialis. Isometrically contract the lower trapezius muscles and pectoralis minor to prevent scapular elevation.

5. Safety factors: In order to avoid elbow hyperextension and undue stress on elbows and wrists, it's probably a good safety precaution to stop short of full elbow extension when performing this exercise. Watch the tendency to elevate and abduct the scapulae. Flex from the hips and avoid spinal flexion and collapsing forward in the seated position. Avoid wrist breaking.

Spotting guidelines: Kneel in front of client, tracking weights with hands.

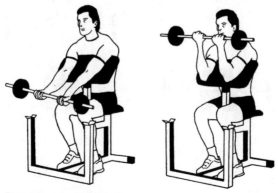

Fig. 10.49–Preacher curl with barbell

Standing Barbell Curl

Equipment used: barbell or EZ curl bar

Moving joints	Joint action	Muscles worked
elbows	flexion	biceps, brachialis, brachioradialis

1. Starting position: Standing, with knees slightly flexed and neutral pelvis, spine, and neck (may be performed with back against a wall). Scapulae are depressed and adducted. Elbows are extended with upper arms tight against body. Palms are supinated with shoulder-width grip, wrists straight.

2. Moving joints: Elbows. All other joints are stabilized, including the knees, pelvis, spine, shoulders, scapulae and wrists.

3. Alignment and technique: Exhale as elbows flex. Keep upper arms pressed against ribs at all times. Lower slowly and with control.

4. Engage and contract the biceps, brachialis, and brachioradialis through both concentric and eccentric phases. Many strength experts recommend a slight pause (isometric contraction) at the top.

5. Safety factors: When weight is too heavy, many clients will rock torso back and forth and swing the weights up (increasing risk of injury to the low back). Keep torso absolutely still and anchor the upper arms against the sides. Watch for wrist breaking. Be sure client goes through full range of motion.

Spotting guidelines: stand in front of client, tracking bar with hands.

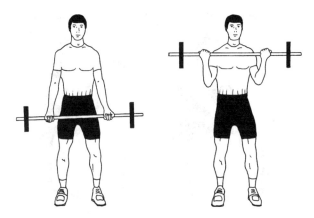

Fig. 10.50–Standing barbell biceps curl

Reverse Curl

Equipment used: dumbbells or barbell (EZ curl may be used), bench

Moving joints	Joint action	Muscles worked
elbows	flexion	biceps, brachialis, brachioradialis

1. Starting position: Assume the same as for barbell curl except that palms are pronated on barbell or dumbbells. This places much more stress on the brachialis. If using dumbbells, exercise may be performed seated.

2-5. See instructions for standing barbell curl.

Hammer Curl

Equipment used: dumbbells, bench

Moving joints	Joint action	Muscles worked
elbows	flexion	biceps, brachialis, brachioradialis

1. Starting position: Assume the same as that for standing barbell curl except that dumbbells are held at sides in mid-pronated position. This places slightly more stress on the brachioradialis. Weights may be lifted simultaneously or alternating. Exercise may be performed seated.

2-5. See instructions for standing barbell curl.

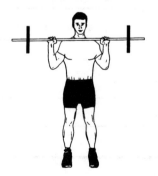
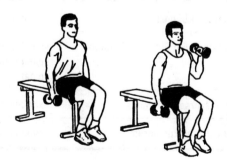

Fig. 10.51–Standing reverse curl with barbell

Fig. 10.52–Seated alternating hammer curl with dumbbells

▼ Exercises for the Abdominals ▼

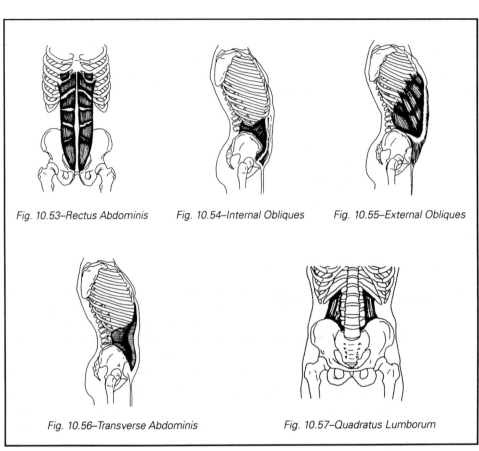

Fig. 10.53–Rectus Abdominis   Fig. 10.54–Internal Obliques   Fig. 10.55–External Obliques

Fig. 10.56–Transverse Abdominis   Fig. 10.57–Quadratus Lumborum

Muscle	Prime Mover for:	Assists with:
Rectus Abdominus	spinal flexion	spinal lateral flexion
Internal and External Obliques	spinal flexion spinal rotation spinal lateral flexion	
Transverse Abdominis	exhalation and expulsion	
Quadratus Lumborum	spinal lateral flexion	

Pelvic Tilt for Abdominals

The pelvic tilt exercise may be used as a beginner exercise to train two muscle groups: the hip extensors (gluteus maximus and hamstrings), and/or the rectus abdominis. When properly performed it is very safe and helps develop body awareness.

Equipment used: mat, slant board

Moving joints	Joint action	Muscles worked
lower spine	lumbar flexion	rectus abdominis
pelvis	posterior pelvic tilt	rectus abdominis

1. Starting position: Lie supine on mat or, for increased resistance, on slant board with hips lower than head. Knees are flexed, feet a comfortable distance from hips, and spine and neck in neutral.

2. Moving joints: Lower spine and pelvis. Try to avoid hip extension and/or pressing into the floor with the feet if the purpose is to work the abdominals. Upper body is relaxed.

3. Alignment and technique: Posteriorly tilt the pelvis through its full range, about 10°, using only the abdominals (this is a small movement); press low back and sacrum to floor. Touch gluteals to see if they are relaxed. Exhale as the pelvis tilts posteriorly and perform a diaphragmatic (abdominal) breath; the abdominal wall should pull in towards the spine on the exhale. Navel should appear to drop in toward floor and should attempt to be lower than the pubic bone. An isometric contraction may be performed at the end of the range of motion.

4. Engage and contract the rectus abdominis. Encourage client to focus on the area between the navel and pubic bone, to feel a tug on the pubic bone from the rectus abdominis.

5. Safety factors: Avoid anteriorly tilting the pelvis and arching the low back. The spine should return only to neutral after the posterior pelvic tilt. Many clients will tend to push with their hip extensors and contract the buttocks; this should be avoided if the purpose is to train the abdominals. Also, many clients will breathe "backwards," and push the abdominal wall out on the exhale. This is an ideal exercise to develop awareness of proper breathing (the abdomen should pull in on the exhale).

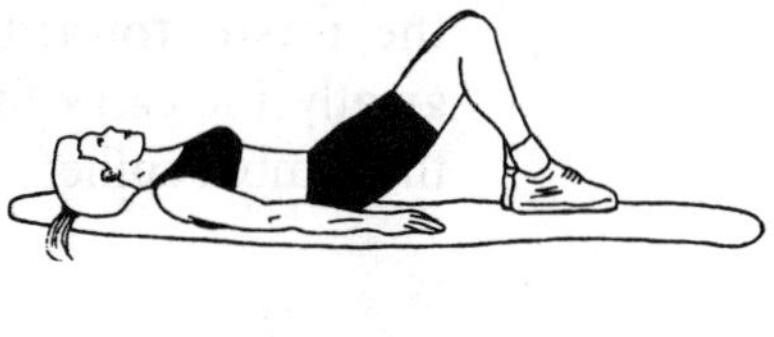

Fig. 10.58–Supine pelvic tilt

Hip Lift

The hip lift (also known as the reverse curl) is simply a more difficult version of the pelvic tilt.

Equipment used: mat, slant board

Moving joints	Joint action	Muscles worked
lower spine	lumbar flexion	rectus abdominis, internal and external obliques
pelvis	posterior pelvic tilt	rectus abdominis

1. Starting position: Lie supine with legs elevated. Hips are flexed at 90° or greater. Knees may be flexed or straight. Hands may be at sides, crossed on chest, behind head, etc.

2. Moving joints: Lower spine and pelvis. Hips are stabilized and kept in one position throughout exercise. Knees are stabilized. Upper spine movement (spinal flexion) increases the difficulty and is optional.

3. Alignment and technique: Posteriorly tilt the pelvis using only the abdominal muscles and curl the lower torso up. Exhale when tilting up and pull the abdominals in (diaphragmatic breath) so that the pubic bone rises higher than the navel. Keep legs and hips locked into a stable position (hip flexors are isometrically contracted). Most clients will only be able to curl the lower torso up about 10°, unless they are very strong and/or have favorable biomechanics (a long torso and flat gluteals help make flexion more visible).

4. Engage and contract the abdominals. Concentrate on pulling the lower area in and feeling a pull on the pubic bone.

5. Safety factors: One of the most common errors is the use of momentum and swinging the legs back and forth to mimic the appearance of a lift. This allows the hip flexors to become the prime movers. Controlled spinal flexion must be performed in order to work the abdominals through full range of motion. Dropping the legs away from the torso (toward the floor) greatly increases the stress on the lumbar spine.

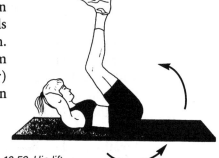

Fig. 10.59–Hip lift

Abdominal Curl (Torso Curl or Crunch)

Equipment used: mat, slant board

Moving joints	Joint action	Muscles worked
lumbar spine	flexion	rectus abdominis, internal and external obliques

1. Starting position: Lie supine (can be inclined for an easier variation, or declined with head lower than spine for a harder variation). Knees are flexed with feet flat on the floor at a comfortable distance from hips (feet may be supported up on a wall or on a bench). Spine and neck are in neutral alignment. Hands and arms may be in a variety of positions (e.g., at the sides, on the chest, fingers behind ears, etc. The closer the hands and arms are to the trunk the easier the lift biomechanically; the longer the lever, the more difficult).

2. Moving joints: Lower spine. Neck should be stabilized in a neutral position and should have no independent movement of its own. To optimally isolate the abdominals, hips should be stabilized.

3. Alignment and technique: Exhale as spinal flexion is performed; use a correct diaphragmatic breath (abdomen pulls in on the exhale). Pull ribs toward pubic bone and pull pubic bone toward ribs (posterior pelvic tilt). Full range of spinal flexion is about 40° (30° with upper torso, 10° with pelvis). Shoulder blades should lift off floor.

4. Engage and contract the abdominals, pulling them in hard on the exhale/lift. Adding an isometric contraction at the top (keep exhaling) increases the difficulty.

5. Safety factors: Avoid jerking or yanking on head or neck; this decreases the effectiveness and increases the risk of injury. Hyperextending the cervical spine (looking at the ceiling while crunching) also places stress on the neck. Many clients do their curl-ups too quickly, using momentum. Keep movements slow and controlled, with focused awareness. Avoid arching the low back as the upper torso is lowered. Supporting feet up on bench (knees flexed at 90°) may be the safest and most comfortable position for clients with a history of back pain.

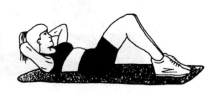

Fig. 10.60–Basic abdominal crunch (hands gently supporting head, feet flat on floor)

Supine Crunch Twist (Rotational Curl-up)

Equipment used: mat, slant board

Moving joints	Joint action	Muscles worked
lower spine	flexion with rotation	internal and external obliques

1. Starting position: Lie supine. There are many variations for both lower and upper body: legs may be elevated, ankles crossed, feet flat on floor, hands behind head, reaching toward legs, etc. Spine and neck are in neutral alignment.

2. Moving joints: Lower spine. Neck is stabilized and has no independent movement. If one or both hands are behind head, shoulder and elbow joints are stabilized (elbow remains in peripheral vision). Lower body is stabilized in order to isolate the obliques.

3. Alignment and technique: Exhale when lifting. Cross one side of upper torso diagonally across toward opposite hip. Shoulder blade lifts up off floor. Movement is slow and controlled.

4. Engage and contract the obliques. Add an isometric contraction at the top to increase the difficulty.

5. Safety factors: Keep hips stabilized on floor and avoid rocking from side to side. As in the basic crunch, avoid yanking on neck. Some clients will perform lots of horizontal shoulder flexion (moving the elbow forward) to mimic the correct action. Avoid momentum.

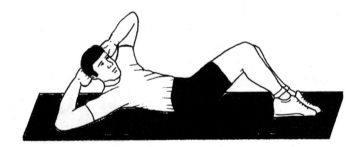

Fig. 10.61–Supine crunch twist

Abdominal Exercise Machines

Many seated "abdominal" machines are designed so that it is much more likely that the exerciser will perform hip flexion instead of spinal flexion. In order to work the abdominals effectively, spinal flexion must be performed through the full range of motion, and the hips must be stabilized.

- Sit so that the axis of rotation, or cam, is aligned with the lower part of the sternum.

- Flex the spine so that the rib cage and pubic bone tilt towards each other. Exhale during flexion, pulling the abdominals in.

Standing Roman Chair

In order to effectively train the abdominals on this apparatus the exerciser needs to already have very strong abdominals as well as good body awareness. A very common mistake that many exercisers make is to perform rapid hip flexion (with either straight or bent knees) with lots of momentum. The correct method is as follows:

- Bring hips in to about 90° of flexion (knees bent) and stabilize them at that degree. This takes a great deal of isometric hip flexor strength.

- Maintaining the isometric contraction of the hip flexors, slowly curl the pubic bone up toward the ribs, exhaling. For most clients, the movement will be small. The moving joint actions are posterior pelvic tilt and lower spinal flexion.

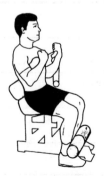
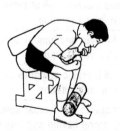
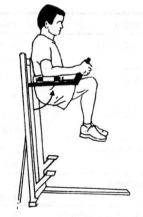

Fig. 10.62–Abdominal machine exercise (trunk curl)   *Fig. 10.63–Standing Roman chair*

▼ Exercises for the Back ▼

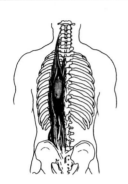

Fig. 10.64–Erector Spinae showing the Longissimus, Spinalis, and Iliocostalis groups

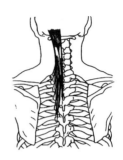

Fig. 10.65–Semispinalis and Multifidus

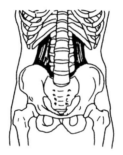

Fig. 10.66–Quadratus Lumborum

Muscle	Prime Mover for:	Assists with:
Longissimus	cervical and thoracic spinal extension, lateral flexion and rotation	
Spinalis	cervical and thoracic spinal extension, lateral flexion and rotation	
Iliocostalis	cervical, thoracic and lumbar spinal extension, lateral flexion and rotation	
Semispinalis	cervical and thoracic spinal extension, lateral flexion and rotation	
Multifidus	cervical, thoracic and lumbar spinal extension, lateral flexion and rotation	
Quadratus Lumborum	spinal lateral flexion	

Seated Back Extension

This may be one of the safer alternatives for mild low back strengthening, especially if the erector spinae muscles contract isometrically as spinal stabilizers and allow the hip extensors to be the prime movers (however, for more effective work, seated back extensions should involve full range of motion trunk extension). Extending (hyperextending) the spine in this exercise is controversial. When recommending low back exercises, make sure you evaluate your client's history of past injury (and physician's recommendations, if any), level of muscular fitness, level of body awareness, and goals.

Equipment used: seated back extension machine

Moving joints	Joint action	Muscles worked
hips	extension	gluteus maximus and hamstrings
lower spine	extension	erector spinae

1. Starting position: Sit with belt across hips, hands on thighs for support. If the goal is to work the hip extensors, align the axis of rotation near the hips. For spinal extensor work, adjust the machine so that the axis of rotation is near the lower thoracic spine.

2. Moving joints: Hips and/or lower spine (depending on goals, etc.). If only hip joint movement is used, spine should be stabilized. Contract the abdominals and maintain neutral spinal alignment throughout the movement. Conversely, hips may be stabilized and spinal movement may be emphasized (in this case, start in spinal flexion, hands on thighs, and move into spinal extension). Neck should be stabilized.

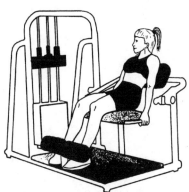

Fig. 10.67–Seated back extension machine exercise (maintain neutral cervical spine)

3. Alignment and technique: Exhale as hips and/or spine extend(s). Movement should be slow and controlled at all times. Return slowly to start, inhaling.

4. Engage and contract the targeted muscle group (gluteus maximus and hamstrings, or erector spinae). Isometrically contract abdominals and erector spinae if hip extensor work is desired. Isometrically contract hip extensors if erector spinae work is the goal.

5. Safety factors: This exercise may be risky for clients with back problems. In this case, discuss appropriate exercises with their physicians. Be conservative, use lighter weight with more repetitions and avoid exercising the low back muscles to failure. Keep neck in a neutral position. Hands should be on thighs when the spine is flexed and weight bearing.

Prone Back Extension

Equipment used: mat

Moving joints	Joint action	Muscles worked
lumbar and thoracic spine	extension	erector spinae

1. Starting position: Lie prone with forehead on mat, and neck in neutral alignment. Hips are pressed into floor, gluteals contracted. For modified cobra, elbows are flexed and pressed into sides, palms on floor. For other variations, arms may be in neutral at sides, or flexed overhead and resting on mat.

2. Moving joints: Lumbar and thoracic spine move. Cervical spinal extensors contract isometrically, maintaining neutral alignment. Hips are stabilized.

3. Alignment and technique: This exercise has several variations. Perhaps the safest and most conservative is the supported, modified cobra position: move smoothly and slowly up onto elbows, hold for a few seconds, and slowly return. Other variations include extending spine with both arms at sides, one arm at side and one arm overhead, both arms overhead, etc. In all cases the extension is smooth and controlled, with pelvis and neck in neutral.

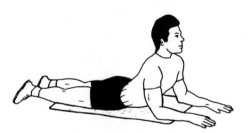

Fig. 10.68–Modified Cobra

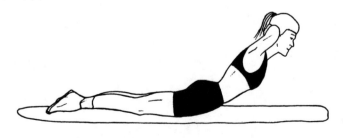

Fig. 10.69–Prone back extension with hands behind head

4. Engage and contract the erector spinae muscles. Isometrically contract the cervical spinal extensors and the buttocks.

5. Safety factors: This exercise may not be appropriate for all clients. If it seems to trigger pain, don't do it (discuss back exercises with the client's physician). Avoid hyperextending the neck; it should have no independent movement.

Back Extension on Roman Chair

This exercise device may be used to work either the hip extensors or the spinal extensors or both, depending on the placement of the hips on the pad.

Equipment used: Roman chair (back extension bench)

Moving joints	Joint action	Muscles worked
lower spine	extension	erector spinae
hips	extension	gluteus maximus, hamstrings

1. Starting position: To isolate the erector spinae, lay over the front pad so that the edge of the pad is slightly above the iliac crest. Flex the spine with head down. As with abdominal crunches, hand position can vary, depending on client goals and muscular strength. Biomechanically, keeping arms at sides is the easiest variation, while arms overhead is the hardest. (For increased hip extensor work, slide hips forward on the front pad so that the edge of the pad is below the iliac crest or even under the upper thighs.)

2. Moving joints: Lower spine. Stabilize hips if the goal is erector spinae strengthening. Cervical spine is stabilized in neutral alignment.

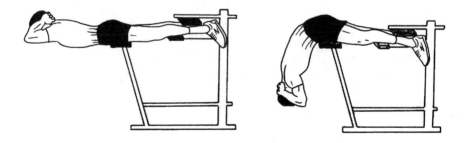

Fig. 10.70–Back and hip extension on Roman chair

3. Alignment and technique: Exhale as spine extends upward. Experts are divided on whether or not the spine should extend just to neutral (parallel to floor), or move beyond neutral into increased extension. All movements, concentric and eccentric, should be very smooth and controlled. Inhale as the spine slowly flexes.

4. Engage and contract the erector spinae muscles. Isometrically contract the cervical spinal extensors and the gluteals and hamstrings.

5. Safety factors: This exercise remains controversial according to several major fitness organizations. Extending the spine up above parallel is especially risky. Carefully consider the client's goals and past history of back problems. Never continue back extension work if it causes pain; and avoid exercising these muscles to failure. Avoid torso swinging, momentum, and sudden, jerky movement. Keep the neck in neutral.

▼ Exercises for the Lower Body ▼

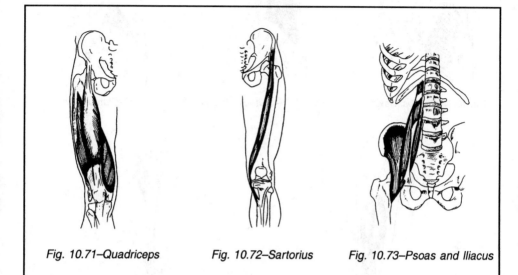

Fig. 10.71–Quadriceps *Fig. 10.72–Sartorius* *Fig. 10.73–Psoas and Iliacus*

Muscle	Prime Mover for:	Assists with:
Quadriceps		
Rectus Femoris	hip flexion and knee extension	
Vastus Lateralis	knee extension	
Vastus Intermedius	knee extension	
Vastus Medialis	knee extension	
Psoas	hip flexion	
Iliacus	hip flexion	
Sartorius		hip flexion
		hip abduction
		hip outward rotation
		knee flexion

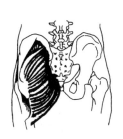

Fig. 10.74–Gluteus Maximus

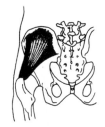

Fig. 10.75–Gluteus Medius

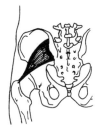

Fig. 10.76–Gluteus Minimus

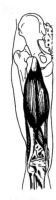

Fig. 10.77–Hamstrings

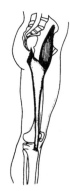

Fig. 10.78–Tensor Fasciae Latae

Muscle	Prime Mover for:	Assists with:
Gluteus Maximus	hip extension hip outward rotation	
Gluteus Medius	hip abduction	
Gluteus Minimus	hip inward rotation	
Hamstrings Biceps Femoris	hip extension knee flexion	
Semitendinosus	hip extension knee flexion	
Semimembranosus	hip extension knee flexion	
Tensor Fasciae Latae		hip abduction, flexion and inward rotation

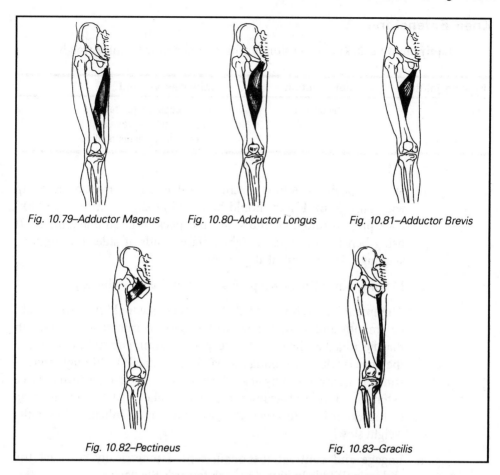

Fig. 10.79–Adductor Magnus   Fig. 10.80–Adductor Longus   Fig. 10.81–Adductor Brevis

Fig. 10.82–Pectineus   Fig. 10.83–Gracilis

Muscle	Prime Mover for:	Assists with:
Adductor Magnus	hip adduction	hip flexion and inward rotation
Adductor Longus	hip adduction	hip flexion and inward rotation
Adductor Brevis	hip adduction	hip flexion and inward rotation
Pectineus	hip adduction hip flexion	inward rotation
Gracilis	hip adduction	hip flexion and inward rotation

Knee Extensions

Equipment used: knee extension machine or bench with ankle weights

Moving joints	Joint action	Muscles worked
knees	extension	quadriceps: rectus femoris vastus lateralis, vastus intermedius, vastus medialis

1. Starting position: Adjust machine so that axis of rotation lines up with knee joint. Knees should be flexed at slightly more than 90°, back pressed into pad, and spine and neck in neutral alignment. If using bench with ankle weights, place hands at sides for support, keeping spine in neutral alignment.

2. Moving joints: Knees. Keep hips, spine and neck stabilized.

3. Alignment and technique: Exhale as knees extend. Movement should be smooth and slow. A one- to two-second isometric contraction may be added at the top. Many experts recommend full extension of the knee (including pulling the patella proximally), although there is some controversy. Physical therapists often use terminal knee extension exercises (flexing the knee only about 10–20° and moving to full extension) to target the vastus medialis. Inhaling, lower the weight slowly.

4. Engage and contract the quadriceps. Isometrically contract the abdominals to help press the back towards the pad.

5. Safety factors: Avoid rapid, jerky, sudden movements that rely on momentum to accomplish the exercise. Watch that the hips and back do not move (as the weight becomes heavy, many clients tend to arch their backs).

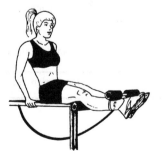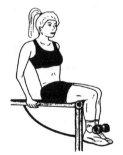

Fig. 10.84–Knee extension machine exercise

Knee Flexion

Equipment used: knee flexion (knee curl) machine

Moving joints	Joint action	Muscles worked
knees	flexion	hamstrings: biceps femoris, semitendinosus, semimembranosus

1. Starting position: May sit, stand, or lie prone, depending on machine. In all cases, hip action should be neutralized. If lying prone on a flat bench, gluteals should be contracted to press hips down and kneecaps should be just off the bench; if standing, neutral pelvis and spine should be maintained. In sitting position, press back, neck and head against pad.

2. Moving joints: Knees. Regardless of position, hips are stabilized without movement, abdominals are isometrically contracted, and neck is in neutral.

3. Alignment and technique: Exhale as knees flex. Bring heels as close as possible to the buttocks. Inhaling, slowly lower.

4. Engage and contract the hamstrings, maintaining contraction through both concentric and eccentric phases.

5. Safety factors: Perhaps the most common error is unnecessary hip movement which can lead to jerking the lower back. Avoid the use of momentum. Keep knees from completely extending.

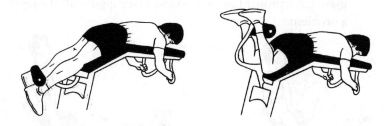

Fig. 10.85–Prone knee flexion

Leg Press or Leg Sled

The leg press movement is similar to a squat; however, because the body is much more supported, it is safer and easier for beginners to learn.

Equipment used: leg press machine

Moving joints	Joint action	Muscles worked
hips	extension	gluteus maximus, hamstrings
knees	extension	quadriceps
ankles	plantar flexion	gastrocnemius, soleus

1. Starting position: Sit, or lie supine (most "supine" machines are actually inclined). Back is pressed flat against pad, neck in neutral. Adjust the seat or the footpad so that the knees are flexed at 90°. Feet should be flat on the footpad.

2. Moving joints: Hips, knees, and ankles. Pelvis is stabilized in neutral; spine and neck do not move. Contract abdominals.

3. Alignment and technique: Exhale as the hips and knees extend. Knees may come to full extension in a controlled manner without hyperextending. Inhale and slowly return to flexion.

4. Engage and contract the gluteus maximus, hamstrings and quadriceps. Isometrically contract the abdominals to maintain the back against the seat.

5. Safety factors: Rapid, uncontrolled movement with knee snapping and jerking increases risk of knee injury. Help clients to feel the difference between full extension of the knee and a forceful "locking" or hyperextending of the knee. Avoid hyperflexion of the knee in a weight bearing position; do not allow the knees to go much beyond 90° of flexion. Avoid arching or flexing the back. Take care to maintain a proper foot position so that slipping off the footpad is not a problem.

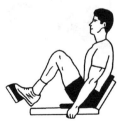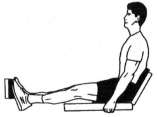
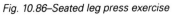

Fig. 10.86–Seated leg press exercise

Squats

The weightroom style squat is an excellent functional exercise; it is needed in activities of daily living, such as lifting heavy objects and getting in and out of chairs. In addition to the ballet style squat, or plié, there are many variations of the weightroom squat, including (from easiest to hardest):

- squat supported by a barre, railing or other fixed object
- unsupported squat over the end of a bench
- unsupported body weight squat (no bench)
- squat with dumbbells resting on thighs
- back squat using Smith press
- back squat using barbell
- front squat using Smith press
- front squat using barbell

Equipment used: may need a barre, bench, dumbbells, barbell, Smith press machine, power rack, etc.

Moving joints	Joint action	Muscles worked
hips	extension	gluteus maximus, hamstrings
knees	extension	quadriceps
ankles	plantar flexion	gastrocnemius, soleus

1. Starting position for back squat: Stand with feet shoulder-width apart, toes straight ahead. Hands have a slightly wider-than-shoulder-width grip (pronated) on the barbell; barbell rests on posterior deltoids (not on base of cervical spine). As lifter stands and takes the full weight on the shoulders, the pelvis, spine, and neck are stabilized in neutral; abdominals are contracted, knees are soft.

2. Moving joints: Hips, knees and ankles. Spine, neck and shoulders must be stabilized in a fixed position without any independent movement during both concentric and eccentric phases.

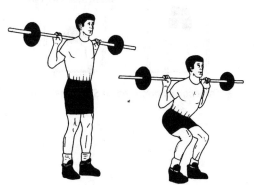

Fig. 10.87–Back squat with barbell

3. Alignment and technique: Inhale as weight is lowered and hips and knees flex. Shift middle third of body (hips and pelvis) back so that knees don't overbend and overshoot the toes. Lower until thighs are almost parallel to floor, keeping torso erect, chest lifted, and head up. Exhale and extend knees and hips, bringing pelvis back into neutral alignment. Lift with legs and buttocks, not back. Keep heels down.

4. Engage and contract the gluteus maximus, hamstrings and quadriceps. Remind your client to be especially conscious on the way up, so as not to lift with the back. Erector spinae and abdominals remain strongly isometrically contracted throughout movement.

5. Safety factors: Always use collars and evenly load the bar. Avoid dropping the hips below the knees as this places tremendous stress on the knee joint. Overshooting the toes with the knee also stresses knee ligaments. Pushing or jerking with the low back should be avoided. Some clients will hunch over and collapse the chest; many clients have a tendency to remain in hip flexion at the top of the movement (contract the buttocks and bring the pelvis into neutral). Watch for proper breathing.

Spotting guidelines: For back squats, stand close behind client without touching. For heavy loads, squat with client and track bar with hands (more than one spotter may be necessary). For front squats, stand in front of client and track bar with hands.

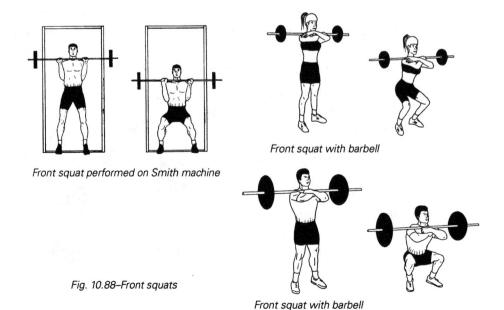

Front squat performed on Smith machine

Front squat with barbell

Fig. 10.88–Front squats

Front squat with barbell

Lunges

The many variations of a lunge include (from easiest to hardest):

- stationary (squat) lunge with wall support
- stationary lunge at Smith press
- step back lunge with wall support
- step back lunge with dumbbells
- forward lunge (back knee bent or back knee straight) onto box or slant board
- forward lunge flat (back knee bent or back knee straight)
- forward lunge with dumbbells, then barbell
- side lunge onto box
- side lunge flat
- side lunge with dumbbells
- crane lunge

Moving joints	Joint action	Muscles worked
hips	extension	gluteus maximus, hamstrings
knees	extension	quadriceps
ankles	plantar flexion	gastrocnemius, soleus

Note: Side lunges require more hip abduction and adduction.

1. Starting position for forward lunge: Stand with knees soft and pelvis, spine and neck in neutral. Dumbbells may be held at sides with palms facing body. Barbell is held in same place as for squats (on posterior deltoids, slightly wider than shoulder width, pronated grip). Feet are shoulder-width apart.

2. Moving joints: Hips, knees and ankles. Torso goes along for the ride, but has no independent movement of its own. Pelvis stays in neutral, as do the spine and neck. Shoulders remain level, head up.

3. Alignment and technique: Lead leg takes big step forward, landing heel first, and flexes knee until the front thigh is parallel to the floor. Front knee should flex no more than 90°; knee should never extend beyond toes. Back knee may be bent at 90° with thigh perpendicular to floor (this is easier), or may be nearly straight with hip fully extended (this takes more balance, coordination, and iliopsoas flexibility). Stay on the ball of the back foot. Torso stays completely upright and stabilized throughout concentric and eccentric phases. Exhale on the return; push off with front foot, balancing, and return

feet to neutral. If balance is difficult, one or two small "stutter" steps are acceptable on the return.

4. Engage and contract the quadriceps, gluteus maximus and hamstrings. Isometrically contract the abdominals, scapular adductors and erector spinae.

5. Safety factors: The lunge is a difficult exercise for many clients (using a slant board or bench is helpful for beginners). Because of the difficulty with balance, coordination, and poor flexibility, a common error is understriding (taking too small a step). This results in the front knee overshooting the toes and creating increased knee stress. Many clients will have difficulty keeping their pelvis neutral as they step forward. The pelvis will tend to tilt anteriorly and the back hip will not be extended (this takes iliopsoas flexibility). Avoid using torso momentum to initiate the backward movement (use the front foot and leg). Back knee should not touch the floor. Watch for hips, knees, and ankles all pointing the same direction; torquing is a common problem.

Spotting guidelines: This is a difficult exercise to spot. For heavy loads, two spotters are recommended, one on either side of client.

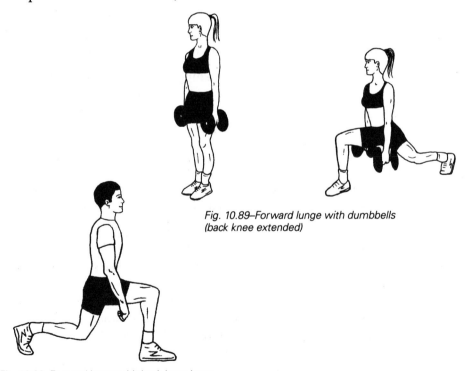

Fig. 10.89–Forward lunge with dumbbells (back knee extended)

Fig. 10.90–Forward lunge with back knee bent

Multi-hip Machine

Many gyms have multi-hip machines that may be used for hip flexor, abductor, adductor, or hip extensor strengthening.

Moving joints	Joint action	Muscles worked
hips	flexion	iliopsoas and quadriceps
	abduction	gluteus medius
	adduction	adductors, gracilis, pectineus
	extension	gluteus maximus, hamstrings

1. Starting position: Stand. Adjust floor pad so that when client stands on it, one hip lines up with the machine's pivot point or axis of rotation. Adjust machine for desired exercise (e.g., hip abduction). Thigh pad should rest against middle part of thigh, and body should be positioned so that the appropriate joint action can be performed through full range of motion. Supporting knee is slightly flexed, while pelvis, spine and neck are in neutral. Hips and shoulders are level.

2. Moving joints: Hips. All other joints are stabilized, including the knees, spine, shoulders and neck. Pelvis maintains neutral pelvic alignment throughout the exercise.

3. Alignment and technique: Exhale as the hip abducts (or flexes, adducts or extends). Move the leg through its full range of motion, lifting it as high as possible within the context of a stable pelvis. There should be no pelvic movement.

4. Engage and contract the prime movers. Isometrically contract the abdominals and the hip and thigh muscles of the support leg (pelvic stabilizers).

5. Safety factors: The most common error is lack of core (pelvic) stabilization. Clients will tend to let their hips move all around and arch their backs. Watch that the support leg maintains a soft, stable knee (knee torque is a common problem), and that shoulders are level. If clients are unable to maintain a neutral stable torso and/or knee, choose an alternative exercise (such as side-lying hip abduction and adduction). Avoid momentum and initiating the movement with the torso. Keep movements slow and controlled.

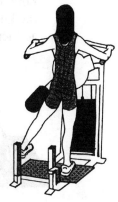

Fig. 10.91—Multi-hip machine standing

Side-lying Hip Abduction and Adduction

Equipment used: mat, ankle weights

Moving joints	Joint action	Muscles worked
hip	abduction	gluteus medius (assisted by the tensor fasciae latae, hip flexors, sartorius and gluteus minimus)
hip	adduction	adductors longus, magnus and brevis, gracilis, and pectineus

1. Starting position: Lie on one side. For abduction: rest head on arm and stack hips. Legs may be extended in a straight line or flexed at the hip about 45°; knees may be extended or flexed depending on the variation. Top arm may be used to stabilize torso. For adduction: rest head on arm and stack hips. Move top leg out of the way of the working bottom leg by flexing the top hip and positioning the top leg so that the hips remain stacked (top leg can rest on a low bench, or knee can be slightly elevated or on the floor, depending on client's hip width and femur length). Bottom (working) leg may have either a flexed or extended knee.

2. Moving joints: Hips. Stabilize knees and ankles. Maintain a stable pelvis and a neutral spine and neck. To best isolate the hip abductors and adductors, stabilize the hips so that no active hip flexion or extension takes place. (Hips may be stabilized in a flexed position, depending on the variation.)

3. Alignment and technique: Move the working leg through its full range of motion, as high as possible without distorting the hips. Keep the knee of the working leg facing forward for both abduction and adduction.

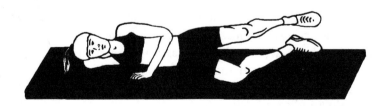

Fig. 10.92–Side-lying hip abduction

4. Engage and contract the hip abductors or the hip adductors, depending on the exercise. Maintain a conscious contraction through both concentric and eccentric phases.

5. Safety factors: The most common error is hips rolling backward or forward; many clients will try to throw the leg up too high, causing the hips to fall out of alignment. Avoid flexing the hips 90° for abduction; this places stress on the gluteus medius tendon. Avoid the "couch potato" position of the neck.

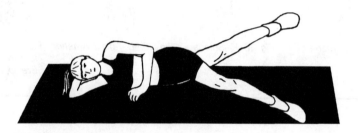

Fig. 10.93–Side-lying hip adduction

▼ Exercises for the Lower Leg ▼

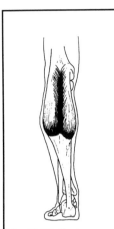

Fig. 10.94–Gastrocnemi

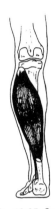

Fig. 10.95–Soleus

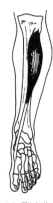

Fig. 10.96–Tibialis Anterior

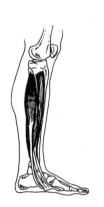

Fig. 10.97–Peroneals
(peroneus Longus,
Brevis, and Tertius)

Muscle	Prime Mover for:	Assists with:
Gastrocnemius	ankle plantar flexion	
Soleus	ankle plantar flexion	
Tibialis Anterior	ankle dorsiflexion ankle inversion	
Tibialis Posterior	ankle inversion	
Peroneus Tertius	ankle dorsiflexion ankle eversion	
Peroneus Longus	ankle eversion	
Peroneus Brevis	ankle eversion	

Heel Raises

Equipment used: step or board, dumbbells or barbell

Moving joints	Joint action	Muscles worked
ankles	plantar flexion	gastrocnemius and soleus

1. Starting position: Stand with feet hip-width distance apart and toes pointing straight ahead. Balls of feet are on the edge of the step or board with heels hanging down. Body is in good standing alignment: knees soft, pelvis, spine and neck neutral, shoulders level. If using dumbbells, hold with mid-pronated grip (palms face sides). If using barbell, rest it across shoulders on the posterior deltoid, hands in pronated, wide grip.

2. Moving joints: Ankles. Entire rest of body should be stabilized with no other joints moving. Although knees are soft, they have no independent movement of their own.

3. Alignment and technique: Exhale and raise up on balls of feet as high as possible. Inhale and slowly lower as far as possible.

4. Engage and contract the gastrocnemius and soleus. Maintain an isometric contraction of the abdominals, quadriceps, etc.

5. Safety factors: Avoid rapid lifting and sudden lowering, which may strain the Achilles tendon. Avoid lowering so far that pain is felt. Watch that the hips and knees stay stable throughout the movement. Balance may be an issue. The exercise may be performed holding onto a rail or wall with no weight or with a weighted belt.

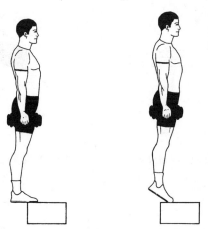

Fig. 10.98–Standing heel raise off a step with dumbbells

Dorsiflexion and Eversion

Equipment used: rubber resistance band, weighted boot, or T-bar device

Moving joints	Joint action	Muscles worked
ankle	dorsiflexion	tibialis anterior, extensor digitorum longus, peroneus tertius
tarsal	eversion	peroneus tertius, peroneus longus, peroneus brevis, extensor digitorum longus

1. Starting position: Sit on floor in proper sitting alignment (spine and neck in neutral, pelvis straight up and down). Hands may be at sides or slightly behind for support; alternatively, client may sit with back against wall. For dorsiflexion, rubber band is placed over top of foot with other end tied to a secure object. For eversion, band is tied in a loop and placed around both feet (feet are hip-width distance apart). Knees are extended without hyper- extension.

2. Moving joints: Ankles and/or tarsal joints. Knees, hips, spine, neck, etc. must be kept stable.

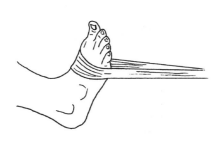

Fig. 10.99–Dorsiflexion with elastic band

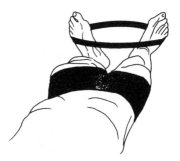

Fig. 10.100–Eversion with elastic band

3. Alignment and technique: For dorsiflexion, pull forefoot toward body as far as possible and slowly return to starting position. For eversion, one or both feet may evert against the resistance of the band (press outside of foot away from midline). An isometric contraction may be added.

4. Engage and contract the dorsiflexors and the everters, respectively.

5. Safety factors: Keep movement smooth and controlled. Avoid locking the knees.

IN SUMMARY

In this chapter, critical information for more than fifty major weightroom exercises was outlined, including the equipment used, what muscles were worked, what joint actions took place, starting position, alignment and technique, safety factors, and spotting tips for each particular exercise.

11

Resistance Training

Designing a Resistance Training Program

When formulating an individualized resistance training exercise prescription, the following steps are helpful:

1. **Determine your clients' short- and long-term goals for muscular fitness.** Do they want to increase strength, muscular endurance, or muscle size (hypertrophy)? Do they want both muscle strength and hypertrophy? Do they want overall general muscle "toning" or body shaping? Are there specific areas of the body in which they want to achieve results?

2. **Identify which muscle groups will be trained.** There are two steps: 1) Create a balanced program that addresses all major muscle groups. Keep in mind that opposing muscle groups and/or muscles on both sides of a joint need to be challenged for muscle symmetry and injury prevention. The major groups include the deltoids, latissimus dorsi, pectorals, scapular adductors, biceps, triceps, abdominals, erector spinae, quadriceps and hamstrings. 2) Add exercises that specifically work client's target areas. For example, if the client wants to focus on abdominals, add exercises that will challenge the abdominals in a variety of ways. For athletes, utilizing the principle of specificity is important: select exercises that train the muscle(s) with the same joint action, range of motion, speed, intensity, and type of contraction that will be needed during the athlete's sport.

3. **Identify areas of injury, or potential injury, that need special attention.** For instance, has your client suffered from back pain in the past? Has he/she had a previous shoulder injury? Does he/she feel a "clicking" and mild pain in the knees when going down stairs? Is there a muscle

imbalance? Does he/she play vigorous singles tennis twice a week? In all these examples, there are resistance exercises that may be helpful and/or should be avoided.

4. **Identify the type of muscle training to be used.** Isometric (good for injured areas and for stabilization training), isotonic (free weights or machines), eccentric (negative training), plyometric, power, or speed training (appropriate for some athletes and sports specific goals) are some options.

5. **Select the specific exercises.** Keep in mind muscle balance, symmetry, the clients' goals and fitness level, and sport specificity if appropriate. Also consider the type of equipment available, whether or not the client will need to take the exercises "on the road" or perform them at home, and whether or not a spotter will be needed.

6. **Select the exercise order.** In general, large muscle groups are worked first. Other options include: core exercises before non-core exercises, alternating push with pull exercises, alternating upper with lower body exercises, and so on.

7. **Determine the frequency of training.** Is your client available to weight train two or three times a week? Does he/she want daily (split routine) training and is he/she committed enough to maintain such a schedule?

8. **Determine the number of sets.** This depends on your client's fitness level, goals and time available for weight training.

9. **Determine the number of repetitions.** The greater the number of repetitions, the lighter the weight (helps develop muscle endurance); the fewer the repetitions, the heavier the weight (enhances muscular strength development).

10. **Determine the intensity (load, or amount of resistance).** There are two major methods for determining the weight load:

    – Trial and error (probably the most common method used for the general public)—find the resistance that your client can lift eight times, but no more than twelve. This method can also be used to determine a client's number of repetition maximums for a particular load, i.e., if an exercise can only be performed six times, that is the six RM load.

    – Percent of 1 RM—this method requires 1 RM (maximal lift) testing in order to figure the desired percentage. For example, if your client can press 100 pounds, 75%, or 75 pounds, would be a good load for the development of both strength and endurance

(10 repetitions). There are charts available with predicted percentage loads and number of repetitions based on a known maximal lift.[72] These charts may also be used to predict the 1 RM based on a client's 10 RM.

11. **Determine the length of the rest period between sets and/or between exercises.** With high intensity training (heavy loads, few repetitions), a longer rest period is generally needed (90+ seconds). With low intensity training (light load, many repetitions), no rest (or a very short rest) may be needed. For sports-specific needs, the rest period may be manipulated to encourage better lactic acid tolerance.

12. **Plan ahead for progressive overload.** For general strength and endurance goals, see the double progressive approach discussed under *Progression* in Chapter 6.

13. **Determine how the training program will be varied over time.** This may be either a within-the-week type variation (e.g., Monday—heavy weights, Wednesday—light weights, Friday—medium to heavy weights), or a longer term type cycling called periodization.

Periodization refers to variations in the training program over the course of several months or a year that help to improve performance and prevent injury, staleness, and burnout. The concept of periodization is supported by Hans Selye's *General Adaptation Syndrome* theory which suggests that the body goes through three phases of adaptation: 1) alarm or shock—muscle soreness develops and performance may decrease as a result of a bout of resistance training; 2) adaptation—the body adapts to resistance training and strength increases; 3) exhaustion or staleness—the body has adapted, reached a plateau, and no new changes take place, or the body is not given a chance to adapt and injury and burnout result. With training variations over time (periodization), staleness, burnout and injury are less likely; the body's potential for increased strength (adaptation to training) is enhanced. According to Fleck and Kraemer, periodization consists of four phases: training for hypertrophy, training for strength, training for power, and training at peak intensity. The whole cycle is followed by a period of active rest (or fifth phase).[72]

The idea behind this type of cycle is to start with high volume (many repetitions and sets), and low intensity. During the following phases, volume is decreased and intensity is increased. However, you can create your own periodization cycle, arranging phases and/or methods of resistance training to suit client needs. Below is a sample program for strength and power development:

Phase	Level	Sets	Repetitions	Weight	Training Methods
1	hypertrophy	4–6	8–20	low weight	high volume training, such as super-sets, giant sets, light to heavy pyramids
2	strength	3–5	3–8	heavy weight	more intense training methods, such as heavy to light pyramids, priority muscle training, full (double) pyramids
3	power	3–5	2–3	heavier weight	more intense training methods utilizing speed
4	peak	1–3	1–3	very heavy weight	blitz training, forced reps, power drills
5	active rest	1–2	8–12	low to moderate weight	circuit weight training, single sets

14. **Evaluate and reassess the program's effectiveness.** This should be an ongoing process; adjustments in the program may need to be made frequently depending on your client's level of motivation, improvement (or lack thereof), level of fatigue or muscle soreness, injuries and interests.

Overcoming strength plateaus

Many clients reach a point where further increases in strength become difficult and progress seems to stop. This is called a plateau. There are several strategies for overcoming strength plateaus, including: choosing different exercises, increasing rest and recovery time, varying the number of sets, repetitions or intensity, and/or choosing a different training system.

Resistance training systems

A knowledge of various systems of resistance training is useful in helping clients to overcome plateaus and optimize results. Varying the method of training can help prevent injuries, overtraining, and boredom. Resistance training systems include:

Single set system—This is the basic, one set of 8–12 repetitions for each muscle group system that is widely recommended and used for beginners and those interested in an effective, time-efficient workout (most of the general public).

Multiple set system—This system is also widely used. It consists of three to six sets of an exercise (usually with the same weight throughout).

Super-set system—A super-set is any combination of two different exercises immediately following one another without a rest (this may be repeated for several sets). This system is popular with bodybuilders and is said anecdotally to produce hypertrophy. There are several different types of super-sets:

- two exercises for the same muscle group: e.g., military press, lateral raises, military press, lateral raises

- two exercises for opposing muscle groups: e.g., military press, lat pull-down, military press, lat pull-down

- two exercises alternating upper body with lower body: e.g., military press, barbell squat, military press, barbell squat

Tri-set system—Tri-sets are similar to super-sets except that three different exercises immediately follow one another (usually for the same muscle group). There is no rest between exercises or between sets. An example might be: barbell incline bench press, flat bench dumbbell fly, standing cable crossovers.

Giant set (also known as a compound set)—These are similar to super-sets and tri-sets except that four to six different exercises may follow one another without a rest. These are often used for muscle groups (such as abdominals) where many different variations of an exercise are possible.

Pyramids—there are three major types of pyramid training:

1. Light to heavy or ascending pyramid (modified DeLorme method)—here the weight is increased and the repetitions decrease with each set.

2. Heavy to light or descending pyramid (two types):
   (a) the Oxford technique, which is simply the reverse of the ascending pyramid above (adjusting for the 1 RM start)—the weight decreases while the repetitions increase, or (b) decreasing weights and decreasing repetitions.

3. Complete pyramid or triangle program—an exhaustive, intense training method combining light-to-heavy with heavy-to-light, first increasing the resistance and then decreasing it.

Pre-exhaustion system—This widely used technique simply means performing exercises that isolate large muscles first, prior to exercises that work both large and small muscles simultaneously. For example, if super-setting bench presses with dumbbell flys, perform the flys first for pre-

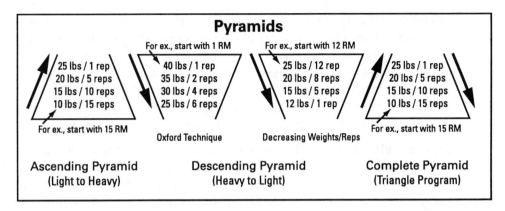

exhaustion of the large pectoralis major and anterior deltoid group. This helps ensure that the smaller triceps group (needed for elbow extension during the bench press) won't fatigue before the larger chest muscles and, thereby, limit the potential for overload.

Priority training—This simple concept entails training weaker, less developed muscles first during workouts while the client is most energetic. Strong, developed muscles are not emphasized, but are put on maintenance during this kind of training.

Split routine system—This is a common method of organizing exercises so that clients can train more frequently during a week. Exercises are arranged so that no body part is worked two days in a row; each muscle group is allowed sufficient recovery time. Because the client weight trains four to six times per week, this system allows for greater volume and higher intensity workouts than would be possible if all exercises were performed together on alternate days.

- four-day split example: Monday/Thursday train legs, gluteals, lower back, and abdominals; Tuesday/Friday train chest, upper back, shoulders and arms.

- six-day split example: Monday/Thursday train lower body (thighs, gluteals and calves); Tuesday/Friday train chest, shoulders and triceps; Wednesday/Saturday train latissimus dorsi, trapezius muscles and biceps.

Blitz system—This intense system is a variation of the split routine. Here a single body part is isolated each day, keeping the duration and volume of the workout the same. Blitz training is often used by bodybuilders and athletes before a competition. For example: Monday—chest, Tuesday—back, Wednesday—shoulders, Thursday—arms, Friday—legs, Saturday—trunk.

Circuit training—Here your client moves quickly from one resistance training exercise to another with very little rest between exercises. Only one set is performed with 8–20 repetitions at 40–60% of 1 RM. The circuit can be repeated several times. Advantages of this system are its time efficiency and the fact that it has also been shown to enhance aerobic conditioning.[73] However, improvements in cardiovascular fitness are substantially less (4–12% increase) than those derived from running-type programs (15–20% increase).

Super-circuit training—This system is growing in popularity for group exercise classes. It alternates approximately three minutes of aerobic-type training (e.g., step aerobics, cycling, treadmill running) with approximately one minute of resistance training for a particular body part. Several different stations or exercises may be used for the resistance training segments.

Partial repetitions (or burn system)—After a set of full range of motion exercises are completed to exhaustion, partial range of motion exercises are performed, also to the point of exhaustion. Strict form must be maintained.

Forced repetitions—Similar to the burn system, forced repetitions are those that are performed after a full set of range of motion exercises are completed to exhaustion. Forced repetitions, however, are assisted. The trainer assists the client to force out additional repetitions with good form and spotting technique.

Eccentric training—Similar to forced repetitions, this type of training emphasizes the "negative" or eccentric phase of the contraction. This can be done with special types of equipment (such as Keiser) in which the resistance can be increased with the push of a button during the eccentric phase, and decreased during the concentric phase; or with the trainer assisting during the concentric phase and allowing your client to lower the weight themselves. Muscles are approximately 30–40% stronger during the eccentric phase, and some studies have shown that eccentric training helps maximize strength and hypertrophy gains.[74] However, it should be noted that eccentric training has also been shown to be a primary instigator of delayed onset muscle soreness and is somewhat controversial.

Super-slow training—In this type of training, repetitions are performed very slowly: concentric contractions may take as long as 10 seconds to move through full range of motion. Once in the fully contracted position, there is a pause (isometric contraction), and then a slow return (about four to six seconds) to the starting position.

Cheat system—Although this system is popular with bodybuilders, it is not recommended because of the high risk of injury. It involves performing a set of exercises to exhaustion, then performing a few more repetitions by breaking good form and allowing momentum and other muscle groups to assist.

Resistance Training Sports

Bodybuilding—Competitive bodybuilders are judged according to muscle hypertrophy, definition and symmetry. Posing ability is also important. A typical bodybuilding routine involves performing several exercises per muscle group to maximize fiber recruitment and stress the muscle from a number of angles. Many sets (four to six) of 8–12 RM are performed with very brief rests (15–45 seconds) between sets. The brief rest periods are said to produce a "muscle pump." Split routines and super-setting are popular training systems. Prior to competition, dietary manipulations are used to reduce body fat.

Power lifting—Power lifters compete in three lifts: the bench press, squat, and the dead lift. The winner must lift the most weight in all three lifts for their weight class. Since the goal is to lift the most weight possible, competitors train for strength with heavy loads (1–6 RM), several sets, and long rest periods (two to five minutes, depending on the resistance). Training revolves around the competition exercises with assistor and stabilizer muscle groups worked last.

Olympic lifting—This Olympic sport involves two events: the snatch and the clean and jerk. The winner totals the most weight between the two lifts for his weight class. Skill and technique are very important in the execution of the lifts. Competitors train for strength and power with heavy loads (1–6 RM), many sets, and lengthy rest periods, with a special emphasis on pulling movements.

Common Training Errors and Mechanisms of Injury

The most common training errors are:

- using too much weight
  (causes poor form and increased risk of injury)

- improper or no warm-up

- loss of core stabilization ability

- not using safety devices

- breath holding (Valsalva maneuver)

- problems with range of motion (too much or not enough)

- performing the exercise too fast

Beginners often:

- have trouble with core and scapular stabilization
- do not know their limits
- need to move slowly to develop kinesthetic awareness
- stop an exercise because of loss of neuromuscular control
- need simple, direct, short cues
- have trouble focusing
- have difficulty telling the difference between muscle soreness and inappropriate joint pain

Intermediates:

- can maintain stability almost all the way through a set
- have better kinesthetic awareness—can isolate muscles
- can perform more complex exercises
- can begin to utilize more advanced training systems
- need more detailed cues
- may plateau

Advanced:

- can maintain stability through entire workout
- can perform sports-specific exercises
- know body well enough to know when to stop
- approach all aspects of workout with patience and thoroughness

Body Part	Common Injuries/ Mechanisms of Injuries	Exercise Example
Cervical spine	ballistic hyperextension	fast full head circles
	ballistic or loaded hyperflexion	yoga plow
Lumbar spine	ballistic hyperextension	Roman chair extensions
		uncontrolled cable hip extensions
	ballistic or loaded extreme flexion	stiff legged dead lifts
		good mornings
	rotation combined with the above	windmills
		bar twists
	hip flexor traction on lumbar spine	bilateral leg lifts
		full sit-ups
Shoulder	impingement	upright rows
		lateral raises with >90° abduction
	rotator cuff problems	behind the neck lat pull-down
		military press
		snatch and power clean
	dislocation	supine DB flys with excess ROM
Knee	hyperflexion	deep squats
		deep lunges

Ergogenic Aids

An ergogenic aid is a substance or device that improves, or is thought to improve, an athlete's performance (some so-called ergogenic aids actually detract from performance). There is a long list of possible ergogenic aids, including: alcohol, drugs, hormones, blood doping, oxygen, vitamins and minerals, carbo-loading, and certain kinds of equipment or clothing. One of the problems with researching the effectiveness of an ergogenic aid is the placebo effect. When an exerciser strongly believes in the benefits of a particular ergogenic aid, this positive thought process can affect the body's response. Following is a brief discussion of several common ergogenic aids.

Anabolic steroids—synthetic derivatives of the male sex hormone testosterone, taken to increase muscle mass and strength. Studies have shown that steroids are effective for this purpose at high dosages[75], but that the risks of taking steroids are very serious. In addition to being illegal and unethical, the risks include: testicular atrophy, reduced sperm count, breast enlargement in men and breast regression in women, prostate gland enlargement in men, masculinization in women, liver damage, cardiovascular disease and personality changes.

Human Growth Hormone (hGH)—a hormone secreted by the pituitary gland, that has been shown to increase lean body mass and decrease fat mass.[76] However, as with steroids, there are several potential risks. These include: acromegaly (broadening of the hands, feet and face, skin thickening, and soft tissue growth), enlargement of internal organs, diabetes, glucose intolerance, hypertension, muscle and joint weakness, and cardiomyopathy leading to death.

Blood doping—an artificial increase in a person's total volume of red blood cells (via transfusion), enhancing endurance performance. Risks include: blood clotting, heart failure, and the potential for improperly labeled blood leading to the transmission of hepatitis and the AIDS virus.

Caffeine—a central nervous system stimulant that is sometimes used to enhance energy levels, endurance, and reaction time. Although not all studies agree, most recent studies show that caffeine does improve endurance performance.[77] Risks include: nervousness, restlessness, insomnia, and tremors in those consuming high doses and/or who are sensitive to caffeine. It also acts as a diuretic, increasing the risk of dehydration and heat stress.

Strength Factors

The influence of genetics on training can scarcely be overemphasized. The goal of proper training is to optimize results within the limits set by each client's genetic potential. In order to avoid unnecessary frustration and discouragement, it is important to help clients understand the following strength factors over which they have no control.

Biomechanical factors

- Limb length—Shorter limbs mean shorter levers, and a shorter lever has a biomechanical advantage (the resistance, or weight, is closer to the fulcrum, or joint, and is easier to lift than a weight that is farther away). In general, clients with shorter limbs will be able to lift more weight than clients with longer limbs, all other factors being equal.

- Tendon insertion—The further the muscle tendon attaches from the joint, or axis, the greater the mechanical advantage affecting muscle strength.

Muscular factors

■ **Muscle belly length**—this is the length of the muscle fibers, not including the attached tendons. Clients with greater muscle tissue (as opposed to tendon, or connective tissue) apparently have a greater ability to develop muscle size and strength.[78]

■ **Muscle fiber composition**—fast twitch (FT) fibers tend to hypertrophy more readily than slow twitch (ST) fibers. (A muscle that hypertrophies increases in fiber size, and strength production is directly related to a muscle's size or cross-sectional area.) Clients who inherited a high percentage of FT fibers will be more successful at strength and power activities, all other factors being equal.

Hormonal factors

■ **Testosterone**—this male sex hormone has a positive influence on the ability of a muscle to hypertrophy; the higher levels of testosterone in men lead to greater muscle size (and greater strength production) and account for the major difference between men and women in strength training. Women typically experience much less muscle growth than men; the average woman has about 1/10 the testosterone of the average man. (Testosterone levels are on a continuum with both men and women; a few women do normally possess higher levels.)

Neurological factors

The most rapid gains in a strength training program are usually at the beginning as the following neurological adaptations take place:

■ recruitment of additional motor units (thus increasing the muscle's ability to produce force)

■ increased synchronization of the motor units (more motor units fire at one time)

■ more efficient recruitment order

■ decreased activity from inhibitory Golgi tendon organs

(*Note:* the factors listed above are not completely under voluntary control)

Overtraining, Detraining and Retraining

Overtraining appears to be caused more by excessive intensity (volume) than by excessive duration or frequency, although there is a wide variation among individual exercisers. Symptoms of overtraining syndrome include:

■ decline in physical performance

- loss of muscle strength, coordination and maximal working capacity
- decreased appetite and body weight loss
- muscle tenderness
- head colds, allergic reactions, or both
- increased number of minor injuries, muscle strains, etc.
- occasional nausea
- sleep disturbances
- elevated resting heart rate
- elevated blood pressure

Several studies have shown that overtraining suppresses normal immune function and causes increased susceptibility to infections.[79] Counseling and complete rest may be necessary to help athletes obsessed with training overcome symptoms. Overtraining syndrome may be avoided by following periodization or cyclical training type programs, alternating hard, easy and moderate periods of training. In addition, allowing adequate time for recovery between bouts of intense exercise is critical.

Detraining is a deconditioning process that occurs as a result of inactivity and/or the cessation of regular physical training. Complete inactivity, or immobilization, causes the most severe responses to detraining. Skeletal muscle atrophy results from inactivity, with a resulting decline in muscle strength and power. However, this decline is relatively small during the first few months, especially if there is no complete immobilization. Several studies have shown that strength can be maintained with only minimal stimulation (exercise once every 10–14 days). In contrast, muscle endurance and cardiorespiratory endurance decrease much more rapidly (two to three weeks of inactivity). This is thought to be due to: decreased oxidative enzyme activities, decreased muscle glycogen storage, disturbance of the acid-base balance, and decreased blood supply to the muscles. Training at least three times per week at 70% of regular training intensity is necessary to maintain cardiorespiratory endurance.[30]

Retraining refers to the concept that the more fit clients are, the more they have to lose during periods of detraining. As a result, they also have more to recover during periods of retraining, and the process of regaining peak fitness will take longer.[30] Retraining, therefore, is influenced by the client's fitness level and the duration of the inactivity.

Giving Clients Feedback

A carefully documented exercise record is invaluable for giving clients feedback about their progress (see sample exercise logs in Appendix B).

Objective information in the form of workloads, heart rates, durations, numbers of sets, etc. should be recorded, as well as more subjective details, such as the client's aches and pains, level of fatigue, comments about workloads, and exercise likes and dislikes. Feedback should be specific and focus on the positive—telling clients specifically what they did well during the previous set is more effective than simply saying "Good job." Appropriate touch may also be a valid way of providing feedback during exercise, helping your client to focus attention on specific target muscles, which may increase exercise effectiveness.[80]

Gender and Age Issues

Women

Women tend to be weaker than men primarily because of their lower quantity of muscle. However, given the same amount of muscle, there are no differences in strength between the sexes.[30] Some studies show that when strength is expressed relative to lean body mass, men are 45% stronger than women in the bench press, but that women are 6% stronger than men in the leg press.[81] The large discrepancy between upper and lower body strength may be due to the fact that both men and women walk, run and climb stairs, but that men usually lift heavy objects with their arms more frequently as compared to women.

Since female muscle tissue has the same physiological characteristics as male muscle tissue, it responds to training in the same manner. Many women are afraid that they will develop large bulky muscles from weight training, but research shows that this is unlikely for the average female. Athletic women who are able to develop significant muscle hypertrophy typically have: 1) higher than normal testosterone levels; 2) a lower than normal estrogen to testosterone ratio; 3) a genetic disposition to develop a greater muscle mass; and 4) a very intense resistance training program.[72] In any event, the principle of reversibility states that all exercise adaptations are transient (temporary) and reversible.

Children

Resistance training for children (especially prepubescent children) has been the subject of controversy in the past due to concerns regarding injury to the epiphyseal growth plates of the long bones. Researchers have reported epiphyseal plate fractures in prepubescent (competitive) weight trainers performing overhead lifts with near maximal resistances. Bone deformation (warping of long bones) has been reported, as have elbow and shoulder epiphyseal injuries resulting from the stress of baseball pitching.[72,30] Below are two sets of guidelines for resistance training for children.

The following information was derived from a 1985 joint workshop with the American Orthopedic Society for Sports Medicine, the American Academy of Pediatrics, the American College of Sports Medicine, the National Strength and Conditioning Association, the National Athletic Trainers Association, the President's Council on Physical Fitness and Sports, the U.S. Olympic Committee, and the Society of Pediatric Orthopedics.

Equipment

1. Strength-training equipment should be of appropriate design to accommodate the size and degree of maturity of the prepubescent.

2. It should be cost-effective.

3. It should be safe, free of defects, and inspected frequently.

4. It should be located in an uncrowded area, free of obstructions, with adequate lighting and ventilation.

Program considerations

1. A preparticipation physical exam is mandatory.

2. The child must have the emotional maturity to accept coaching and instruction.

3. There must be adequate supervision by coaches who are knowledgeable about strength training and the special problems of prepubescents.

4. Strength training should be a part of an overall comprehensive program designed to increase motor skills and level of fitness.

5. Strength training should be preceded by a warm-up period and followed by a cool-down period.

6. Emphasis should be on dynamic concentric contractions.

7. All exercises should be carried through a full range of motion.

8. Competition is prohibited.

9. No maximum lift should ever be attempted.

Prescribed program

1. Training is recommended two or three times a week for 20- to 30- minute periods.

2. No resistance should be applied until proper form is demonstrated. Six to 15 repetitions equal one set; one to three sets per exercise should be performed.

3. Weight or resistance is increased in one- to three-pound increments after the prepubescent performs 15 repetitions in good form.

The following was developed based on information from the book *Strength Training for Young Athletes* by Kraemer, W. J., and Fleck, S. J. Human Kinetics Publishers, Champaign, IL, 1993.

Age	Considerations
7 or younger	Introduce child to basic exercises with little or no weight; develop the concept of a training session; teach exercise techniques; progress from body weight calisthenics, partner exercises, and lightly resisted exercises; keep volume low.
8–10	Gradually increase the number of exercises; practice exercise technique in all lifts; start gradual progressive loading of exercises; keep exercises simple; gradually increase training volume; carefully monitor toleration to the exercise stress.
11–13	Teach all basic exercise techniques; continue progressive loading of each exercise; emphasize exercise techniques; introduce more advanced exercises with little or no resistance.
14–15	Progress to more advanced youth programs in resistance exercise; add sport-specific components; emphasize exercise techniques; increase volume.
16 or older	Move child to entry-level adult programs after all background knowledge has been mastered and a basic level of training experience has been gained.

Note: If a child of any age begins a program with no previous experience, start the child at previous levels and move him or her to more advanced levels as exercise toleration, skill, amount of training time, and understanding permit.

For additional information, see the National Strength and Conditioning Association's 1985 position paper on Prepubescent Strength Training.[82]

Seniors

Both the number and the size of muscle fibers (especially fast twitch) decrease with age; this appears to be accompanied by a reduced ability of the nervous system to process information and excite muscles. These factors, along with an increasingly sedentary, inactive lifestyle, account for the decreases in muscle strength found in seniors. These decreases can be dramatic; one study found that 92% of males and females age 40–60 could easily open a jar, but in people age 71–80, only 32% could open the jar.[83] Decreased muscle strength and muscle atrophy are related to decreased metabolism, increased body fat (creeping obesity), decreased bone density, and decreased ability to perform everyday activities.

Fortunately, some of these "effects of aging" appear to be modifiable with appropriate strength training. Studies on 90-year-old subjects training at intensities as high as 80% of 1 RM have shown dramatic changes in strength and muscle hypertrophy.[84]

ACSM Guidelines for Resistance Training for Healthy Older Adults

Intensity	A minimum of one set each of 8–10 exercises involving the major muscle groups with each set involving 8–12 repetitions that elicit a perceived exertion rating of 12–13 (somewhat hard)
Frequency	Performed a minimum of two days per week, resting a minimum of 48 hours between sessions
Duration	Sessions lasting more than 60 minutes may have a detrimental effect on exercise adherence. Ideally a total body resistance training session should be completed within 20–30 minutes

IN SUMMARY

In this chapter, steps for creating an individualized resistance training exercise prescription were discussed. Periodization and plateaus were defined, and several different resistance training systems were described. Common training errors and mechanisms of inquiry were covered. Some popular ergogenic aids were briefly discussed. Factors influencing strength were listed, and principles of overtraining, detraining, and retraining were described. Strength training, as it relates to special concerns of women, children, and seniors, was discussed.

Chapter 12

Business Aspects and Professional Responsibilities

Getting Started

1. Develop your business plan

This can include a personal mission statement that defines your personal goals and code of ethics, and/or your professional and financial goals. Where would you like your business to be in a year, five years, or ten years? How many clients would you like to have? How much money do you want to make? How much time and energy do you want to commit? Do you want to eventually hire other trainers? Write down the steps you will need to take to meet your goals, and develop a timeline for completing those steps.

2. Determine your target market

Do you prefer working with men or women? Are you interested in working with youth, young professionals, blue collar workers, executives, mid-life clients, or seniors? Perhaps your expertise is in working with special needs clients: handicapped, post-rehabilitation, pregnant, diabetic, or overweight. Do you prefer athletes, bodybuilders, or the deconditioned, harder-to-motivate client? Determining your target market will affect your marketing strategies.

3. Develop your marketing plan

Choose professional-looking business cards, stationary, and resume. You may want to formulate a business name and/or logo; the services of a graphic designer can be valuable in helping to devise a business look and identity that is truly yours. Many trainers also develop an advertising brochure that lists their services and qualifications.

233

Decide how you will attract your target market. For instance, if your target market consists of clients with special needs, networking with physicians (e.g., orthopedists, cardiologists and rheumatologists) and physical therapists may help you get referrals. In addition, OB-GYNs may be willing to refer their pregnant or post-natal patients to you, if that is your specialty client focus. (When approaching physicians, be organized and concise. Describe your credentials, explain what you can do for their patients and ask if you may leave your cards, brochures or flyers in the office waiting room.) Consider what your target clients do, what organizations they may belong to, what papers they may read, what places they may frequent, and so on. Below are additional strategies for attracting clients.

- Network with other health care professionals. Set up referral networks with massage therapists, dietitians, nutritionists, psychotherapists, social workers, registered nurses and chiropractors.

- Network with equipment stores. Small, independent, equipment-only stores are often open to developing relationships with trainers. This may include referrals for training sessions, free consultations for customers who spend a certain amount of money in the store, or allowing you to leave your brochures in a visible place.

- Speak for local organizations. Volunteer your expertise at the Rotary Club, National Association of Women Business Owners, church groups, social clubs, support groups, and other community associations. Look through the telephone book's yellow pages to see what organizations are nearby. Most groups appreciate a generalized presentation on such subjects as the benefits of exercise, how to incorporate exercise into your daily life, travel and exercise, and getting started with a walking program. This would not be the time to make a sales pitch, but if you speak in a professional manner and you are informative, people will listen and want to know more (have your brochures and business cards available).

- Write fitness and health articles for newspapers and/or have a fitness message on the radio as part of a station's regular programming. Write news releases on such noteworthy occasions as attending a major conference, hiring a new trainer, or expanding to new locations. Send these releases to fitness and health writers at a variety of local papers and periodicals and follow up a week later.

- Use word of mouth. Offer your current clients a free session or two for every person they refer who starts a training program. You may also consider offering a free session to visible professionals, such as hairdressers, hotel concierges and journalists, in exchange for referrals.

■ Offer gift certificates to existing clients that they can use as gifts for friends (these can also be advertised in your flyers or brochures).

■ Direct mail your flyers and/or distribute them in parking lots, stores and health clubs. Direct mail can be expensive (figure the cost of a mailing list and stamps, plus the cost of your flyers), but may be a valuable source of clients.

4. Decide if you will be an employee or an independent contractor

If you work for a club, you may be either an employee or an independent contractor; if you are self-employed, you are probably an independent contractor. Independent contractors are responsible for their own taxes, benefits, training, etc. Employees have their taxes deducted, and may be eligible for benefits and training.

Self-employment brings with it many business decisions, especially how the business will operate and under what form. There are three main choices for you to consider: 1) corporate, 2) partnership, or 3) sole proprietorship. Because there are various pros and cons addressing all of these business choices, AFAA recommends that you acquire the book *Legal Aspects of Personal Fitness Training* by Brian E. Koeberle, JD. To order, write to Professional Reports Corporation, 4571 Stephen Circle, N.W., Canton, Ohio 44718-3629 or call (800) 336-0083. You should also seek legal counsel prior to establishing your business.

5. Obtain appropriate licenses and/or insurance

After you have decided whether to run your business as a sole proprietorship (you and your business are the same financial entity), a partnership (two or more people share profits and losses), or a corporation (a legal entity independent of the owners), you will need to obtain several licenses and permits, depending on where you live. At the county clerk's office inquire about: a business license, a state sales tax license, and registering your business name. You will probably need to set up a business checking account. Always carry liability insurance. Reasonable group policies for instructors are offered by AFAA and other organizations.

6. Establish your business policies

Rates for personal training vary according to where you live. In general, the closer you are to a metropolitan area, the higher the rate. The best way to determine how much you will charge is to find out what other trainers in the area are charging and decide on a similar fee. Also, it is fairly common for trainers to discount when several sessions are purchased in advance (e.g., a client can buy 10 sessions for the price of eight). Set clear policies regarding how and when your clients should pay for their personal training. (Note: State law may impact what services can be sold in advance of service provision. Personal fitness trainers should consult with their individual legal counsel to learn what they can do in this regard.)

Offer a free trial session, fitness assessment, or consultation. Many trainers offer a free initial session of some type to help attract clients. Again, it may be worthwhile to see what your competition offers, if anything.

You should inform clients of the cancellation and late policies at their first session. Typically, clients pay for sessions canceled with less than a 12-hour notice. It is a good idea to also put such policies in writing.

(Note: State law may require that some of these policies be posted in a very visible place. Individual legal counsel should be consulted as to such matters.)

7. **Decide what equipment you will need and other expenses you may incur**
   This list may include:
    1. answering machine
    2. pager
    3. personal computer with personal trainer software
    4. professional clothing
    5. professional journals
    6. textbooks
    7. tapes and videos
    8. professional memberships
    9. continuing education
    10. advertising
    11. business licenses and insurance
    12. travel and use of own car
    13. office expenses
    14. bookkeeping service
    15. taxes
    16. home gym for training clients
    17. portable exercise equipment (e.g., rubber tubing, step, slide, ankle weights, light handweights, pedometer, jump rope, water resistance equipment, weight belt and/or weightroom gloves, mat, towel and clipboard)

18. fitness assessment equipment (e.g., blood pressure cuff and stethoscope*, skinfold calipers, tape measures, heart rate monitor, step box, sit and reach box, mat and stopwatch)

19. emergency response plan and procedures

20. appropriate first aid equipment and supplies

*In some states, blood pressure may only be taken by a licensed health care provider. Always check with the given state's laws and regulations before taking vital signs.

Determining Your Professional Capability

What are the qualities that you would want in a personal fitness trainer? They might include:

■ having a thorough knowledge base in exercise, health and fitness

■ being certified

■ taking continuing education seriously

■ behaving professionally

■ being a good leader

■ having a suitable personality

■ being genuinely interested in helping others

■ being a good role model

■ adhering to all applicable laws and regulations

■ avoid overstepping professional competency and entering a field or domain reserved for licensed professionals

Now make your own list and strive to be the very best you can be.

Continuing Your Education

Since the fitness industry interfaces with the scientific, research and medical communities, it is a given that fitness guidelines and information are going to change over time. It is critical that you continue reading, attending seminars, workshops and conferences, and networking with other health care professionals on a regular basis in order to remain professionally competent and to be your best. Below are some suggestions for educational growth.

■ **Return to school.** The reality is, especially in the medical community, that degrees convey credibility and knowledge. And knowledge is power!

■ **Attend higher level workshops and conferences.** Most of the major fitness organizations now provide appropriate seminars on a variety of topics.

■ **Go on for advanced certifications.** Again, most major fitness organizations offer a "higher level" test of your competency.

■ **Subscribe to (and read) as many professional journals** as you can (see the suggested list of journals and magazines in Appendix A).

■ **Read textbooks** (see Appendix A).

■ **Learn to read research.** Reading research in quality, peer-reviewed journals will teach you to think scientifically. Critical, objective thinking is important in a field in which myths abound and naive or misinformed clients are always trying to find a "magic pill or formula" to help them achieve their goals more easily.

Staying within Your Scope of Practice

Recognize the limits of your knowledge and expertise. It is not appropriate (and may even be illegal) for you, the personal fitness trainer, to manipulate client's bodies, diagnose injuries or physical complaints, give specific dietary advice, perform maximal stress tests, or provide psychological counseling unless you have additional training and qualifications (and, under some circumstances, state licensing) in these areas.

Remember, a personal fitness trainer is a skilled teacher, motivator, communicator, and continual student of fitness and positive lifestyle change. Trainers serve a valuable purpose in helping people become healthier and happier, and in improving the quality of many lives.

IN SUMMARY

In this section, various aspects of developing a personal training business, from marketing to insurance to pricing, were briefly discussed. A list of potential expenses was provided as well as suggestions for growing as a trainer and continuing your education. Staying within your scope of practice was emphasized.

References

1. American Heart Association. *1989 Heart facts.* Dallas: American Heart Association, 1989.

2. Boring, C. C., T.S. Squires, and T. Tong. Cancer statistics, 1992. *Cancer.* 42.1 (1992): 19-38.

3. Ballard-Barbash, R., et al. Physical activity and risk of large bowel cancer in The Framingham Study. *Cancer Res.* 50.12 (1990): 3610-3613.

4. Helmrich, S. P., et al. Physical activity and reduced occurrence of non-insulin dependent diabetes mellitus. *N. Engl. J. of Med.* 325 (1990): 147-152.

5. Dalsky, G. P. The role of exercise in the prevention of osteoporosis. *Comp. Ther.* 15 (1989): 30-37.

6. Cypress, B. K. Characteristics of physician visits for back symptoms: a national perspective. *Am. J. of Public Health* 73 (1983): 389-395.

7. Stephens, T., D.R. Jacobs Jr., and C.C. White. A descriptive epidemiology of leisure-time physical activity. *Public Health Rep.* 100 (1985): 147-158.

8. Van Itallie, T. B. Health implications of overweight and obesity in the United States. *Ann. Intern. Med.* 103 (1985): 983-988.

9. Bray, G. A. and D.S. Bray. Obesity, I: pathogenesis. *West. J. of Med.* 149 (1988): 429-441.

10. van Dale, D. and W.H.M. Saris. Repetitive weight loss and weight regain: effects on weight reduction, resting metabolic rate, lipolytic activity before and after exercise and/or diet treatment. *Am. J. of Clin. Nutr.* 49 (1989): 409-416.

11. Mattson, M. E., E.S. Pollack, and J.W. Cullen. What are the odds that smoking will kill you? *Am. J. of Public Health* 77 (1987): 425-431.

12. Dembroski, T., et al. Components of hostility as predictors of sudden death and myocardial infarction in the multiple risk factor intervention trial. *Psychosom. Med.* 51 (1989): 514-522.

13. American College of Sports Medicine. 2000. *Guidelines for exercise testing and prescription.* 6th ed. Baltimore, MD: Lippincott Williams & Wilkins.

14. American College of Obstetricians and Gynecologists. *Exercise during pregnancy and the postpartum period.* (Technical Bulletin #189). Washington, DC: American College of Obstetricians and Gynecologists, 1994.

15. Herbert, D.L. and W.G. Herbert. *Legal aspects of preventive and rehabilitative exercise programs.* 2nd ed. Canton: Professional Reports Corp.

16. Golding, L.A., C.R. Meyers, and W. E. Sinning. *Y's way to physical fitness: complete guide to fitness testing and instruction.* 3rd ed. Champaign: Human Kinetics Pub, 1989.

17. The fifth report of the Joint National Committee on Detection, Evaluation and Treatment of High Blood Pressure (JNCV). *Arch. of Intern. Med.* 153 (1993): 154-183.

18. Lohman, T., A.F. Roche, and R. Martorell. Eds. *Anthropometric standardization reference manual.* Champaign: Human Kinetics Pub, 1988.

19. Durnin, J.V.G.A. and J. Womersey. Body fat assessed from total body density and its estimation from skinfold thicknesses: measurements on 481 men and women aged 16-72 years. *Br. J. of Nutr.* 32 (1974): 77-97.

20. Jackson, A. S. and M.L. Pollock. Generalized equations for predicting body density of men and women. *Br. J. of Nutr.* 40 (1978): 407-504.

21. Millar, W.J. and T. Stephens. The prevalence of overweight and obesity in Britain, Canada, and the United States. *Am. J. of Public Health* 77 (1987): 38-41.

22. Blair, S.N., H.W. Kohl, R.S. Paffenbarger, et al. Physical fitness and all cause mortality: a prospective study of healthy men and women. *JAMA* 262 (1989): 2395-2401.

23. McArdle, W.D., F.I. Katch, and V.L. Katch. *Exercise physiology, energy, nutrition and performance.* 3rd ed. Philadelphia: Lea & Febiger, 1990.

24. Kline, G.M., J.P. Porcari, R. Hintermeister, et al. Estimation of VO_2 max from a one-mile track walk, gender, age, and body weight. *Med. Sci. Sports and Exer.* 19 (1987): 253-259.

25. Fitness & Amateur Sport Canada. *Canadian standardized test of fitness operations manual.* 3rd ed. Ottawa: Fitness & Amateur Sport Canada.

26. Gettman, L.R. Fitness testing. *Resource manual for guidelines for exercise testing and prescription.* Eds. S. Blair, P. Painter, R. Pate, et al. Philadelphia, PA: Lea & Febiger, 1988. 168.

27. Melleby, A. *The Y's way to a healthy back.* Piscataway: New Century Pub, 1982.

28. American College of Sports Medicine. The recommended quantity and quality of exercise for developing and maintaining cardiorespiratory and muscular fitness in healthy adults. (Position Stand). *Med. Sci. Sports and Exer.* 22.2 (1990): 265-274.

29. Pollock, M.L. and J.H. Wilmore. *Exercise in health and disease: evaluation and prescription for prevention and rehabilitation.* 2nd ed. Philadelphia: W. B. Saunders, Co., 1990.

30. Wilmore, J.H. and D.L. Costill. *Physiology of sport and exercise.* Champaign: Human Kinetics Pub., 1994.

31. Hettinger, R. *Physiology of strength.* Springfield: Charles C. Thomas, 1961.

32. Graves, J.E., M.L. Pollock, A.E. Jones, et al. Specificity of limited range of motion variable resistance training. *Med. Sci. Sports and Exer.* 21 (1989): 84-89.

33. Braith, R.W., J.E. Graves, M.L. Pollock, et al. Comparison of two versus three days per week of variable resistance training during 10 and 18 week programs. *Int. J. of Sports Med.* 10 (1989): 450-454.

34. de Vries, H.A. Quantitative electromyographic investigation of the spasm theory of muscle pain. *Am. J. of Phys. Med.* 45.3 (1966): 119-134.

35. Knott, M. and D.E. Voss. *Proprioceptive neuromuscular facilitation.* New York: Harper & Row, 1968.

36. McAtee, R.E. *Facilitated stretching.* Champaign: Human Kinetics Pub., 1993.

37. Margen, S. and Editor of UC Berkeley Wellness Letter. *The wellness encyclopedia of food and nutrition.* New York: Health Letter Assoc, 1992.

38. Expert Panel of the National Cholesterol Education Program. Report of the NCEP expert panel on detection, evaluation, and treatment of high blood cholesterol in adults. *Arch. of Int. Med.* 148 (1988): 36-39.

39. Grundy, S.M. Dietary therapy for different forms of hyperlipoproteinemia. *Circulation* 76 (1987): 523-528.

40. Harris, W.S. Can fish oil retard atherosclerosis? *Practical Cardiology* 15 (1989): 25-32.

41. Nishimune, T., T. Yakushiji, T. Sumimoto, et al. Glycemic response and fiber content of some foods. *Am. J. of Clin. Nutr.* 54.2 (1991): 414-419.

42. Coyle, E.F. and E. Coyle. Carbohydrates that speed recovery from training. *Phys. and Sports Med.* 21.2 (1993): 111-123.

43. Clark, N. Carbohydrates: the complexities of a simple food. *Phys. and Sports Med.* 21.6 (1993): 49-55.

44. Clark, N. *Sports nutrition guidebook.* Champaign: Human Kinetics Pub., 1990.

45. Reynolds, R.D. Vitamin supplements: current controversies. *J. of the Am. Coll. of Nutr.* 13 (1994): 118-126.

46. Brooks, G. *Antioxidants and the elite athlete.* (Paper). Dallas: Read before the 39th annual meeting of the ACSM. May 27,1992.

47. Kleiner, S.M. Supplement Savvy. *Phys. and Sports Med.* 22.8 (1994): 29-30.

48. Burckes-Miller, M. and D. Black. Male and female college athletes: prevalence of anorexia nervosa and bulimia nervosa. *Athl. Training* 23 (1988): 137-140.

49. Kuczmarski, R.J., K.M. Flegal, S.M. Campbell, and C.L. Johnson. The increasing prevalence of overweight among US adults. The National Health and Nutrition Examination Surveys, 1960 to 1991. *JAMA* 272 (1994): 205-211.

50. Kumanyika, S. Obesity and black women. *Epidemiol. Rev.* 9 (1987): 31-50.

51. Elliot, D.L., et al. The sustained decrement in resting metabolic rates following massive weight loss. *Am. J. of Clin. Nutr.* 49 (1989): 93-96.

52. King, A.C., et al. Diet vs. exercise in weight maintenance. *Arch. of Intern. Med.* 149 (1989): 2741-2746.

53. Clark, N. How to gain weight healthfully. *Phys. and Sports* Med. 19.9 (1991): 53-54.

54. Bandura, A. *Social learning theory.* Englewood Cliffs: Prentice Hall, 1977.

55. Taylor, C.B., N.H. Miller, and J. Flora. Principles of health behavior change. *Resource manual for guidelines for exercise testing and prescription.* Ed. ACSM. Philadelphia: Lea & Febiger, 1988.

56. Stephens, T. Secular trends in adult physical activity: exercise boom or bust? *Res. Q. in Exerc. and Sport* 58 (1987): 94-105.

57. Dishman, R.K. *Overview. Exercise adherence.* Ed. R.K. Dishman. Champaign: Human Kinetics Pub., 1988.

58. Dishman, R.K. *Advances in exercise adherence.* Champaign: Human Kinetics Pub., 1994.

59. Rogers, C.R., E.T. Gendlin, D.J. Keisler, and C.D. Truax. *The therapeutic relationship and its impact.* Madison: University of Wisconsin Press, 1967.

60. Gavin, J. and N. Gavin. *Psychology for health fitness professionals.* Champaign: Human Kinetics Pub., 1995.

61. Jampolsky, G.G. *Love is letting go of fear.* Berkeley: Celestial Arts, 1979.

62. Walsh, D.J. and J.C. Fernyhough. Back injury management. *Rehab. Mgmt.* 8.3 (1995): 30-34.

63. Cailliet, R. *Low back pain syndrome.* 3rd ed. Philadelphia: F.A. Davis, 1995.

64. Artal Mittelmark, R., R.A. Wiswell, and B.L. Drinkwater, eds. *Exercise in pregnancy.* Baltimore: Williams and Wilkins, 1991.

65. Lokey, E.A., Z.V. Tran, C.L. Wells, et al. Effects of physical exercise on pregnancy outcomes; a meta-analytic review. *Med. Sci. and Sports Exerc.* 23 (1991): 1234-1239.

66. Tafari, N., R.L. Naege, and A. Gobzie. Effects of maternal undernutrition and heavy physical work during pregnancy on birth weight. *Br. J. of Obstet. Gyn.* 87 (1980): 222-226.

67. Milunsky, A., M. Ulcickas, K. Rothman, et al. Maternal heat exposure and neural tube defects. *JAMA*, 268 (1992): 882-885.

68. McMurray, R.G., M.F. Mottola, L.A. Wolfe, et al. Recent advances in understanding maternal and fetal responses to exercise. *Med. Sci. Sports Exerc.* 25.12 (1993): 1305-1321.

69. Evans, W. and I. Rosenberg. *Biomarkers: the 10 determinants of aging you can control.* New York: Simon & Schuster, 1991.

70. Heath, G.W. Exercise programming for the older adult. *Resource manual for guidelines for exercise testing and prescription.* Ed. ACSM. Philadelphia: Lea & Febiger, 1988.

71. American Association of Cardiovascular and Pulmonary Rehabilitation. *Guidelines for cardiac rehabilitation programs.* Champaign: Human Kinetics Pub., 1991.

72. Fleck, S.J. and W.J. Kraemer. *Designing resistance training programs.* Champaign: Human Kinetics Pub., 1987. 62.

73. Gettman, L.R. and M.L. Pollock. Circuit weight training: a critical review of its physiological benefits. *Phys. and Sports Med.* 9 (1981): 44-60.

74. Dudley, G.A., P.A. Tesch, B.J. Miller, and P. Buchanan. Importance of eccentric actions in performance adaptations to resistance training. *Aviation, Space, Env. Med.* 62 (1991): 543-550.

75. Forbes, G.B. The effect of anabolic steriods on lean body mass: the dose response curve. *Metabolism* 34 (1985): 571-573.

76. Rudman, D., A.G. Feller, H.S. Nagraj, et al. Effects of human growth hormone in men over 60 years old. *New Eng. J. of Med.* 323 (1900): 1-6.

77. Dodd, S.L., R.A. Herb, and S.K. Powers. Caffeine and exercise performance: an update. *Sports Med.* 15 (1993): 14-23.

78. Westcott, W. *Strength Fitness.* 3rd ed. Dubuque: W. C. Brown, Pub., 1991.

79. Kuipers, H. and H.A. Keizer. Overtraining in elite athletes: review and directions for the future. *Sports Med.* 6 (1988): 79-92.

80. Rothenberg, B. and O. Rothenberg. *Touch training for strength.* Champaign: Human Kinetics Pub., 1995.

81. Wilmore, J.H. Alterations in strength, body composition, and anthropometric measurements consequent to a 10-week weight training program. *Med. Sci. Sports and Exer.* 6 (1974): 133-138.

82. National Strength and Conditioning Association. Prepubescent strength training. (Position Paper). *Nat. Str. and Cond. J.* 7 (1985): 27-31.

83. Saltin, B. *Aging, health and exercise performance*. (Provost Lecture Series). Muncie: Ball State University, 1990.

84. Fiatarone, M.A., E.C. Marks, N.D. Ryan, et al. High intensity strength training in nonagenarians: effect on skeletal muscle. *JAMA*. 263 (1990): 3029-3034.

85. Blair, S.N., J. Shaten, K.D. Brownell, et al. Body weight change, all cause mortality, and cause-specific mortality in the multiple risk factor intervention trial. *Ann. Intern. Med.* 119 (1993): 749-757.

86. Baechle, T.R. *Essentials of strength training and conditioning*. Champaign: Human Kinetics Pub., 1994.

87. Pate, R., M. Pratt, S. Blair, et al. Physical activity and public health: a recommendation from the Centers for Disease Control and Prevention and the American College of Sports Medicine. *JAMA*. 273 (1995): 402-407.

88. Chu, D.A. *Explosive power and strength: complex training for maximum results*. Champaign: Human Kinetics Pub., 1996.

89. Centers for Disease Control and Prevention. *Physical activity and health at-a-glance*. A report from the Surgeon General. Atlanta: Centers for Disease Control and Prevention, 1996.

90. Campbell, W., M. Crim, et al. Increased energy requirements and changes in body composition with resistance training in older adults.1-4 *American Journal of Clinical Nutrition*. 60 (1994): 167-75.

91. Hurley, B. Does strength training improve health status? *Strength and Conditioning*. 6 (1994): 7-13.

92. Melby, C., C. Scholl, et al. Effect of acute resistance exercise on postexercise energy expenditure and resting metabolic rate. *The American Physiological Society*. 0161-7567/93 (1993): 1847-1853.

93. Messier, S. and E. Dill. Alterations in strength and maximal oxygen uptake consequent to Nautilus circuit weight training. *Research Quarterly for Exercise and Sport*. 56.4 (1985): 345-351.

94. Westcott, W. and J. Guy. A physical evolution. *IDEA Today*. October 1996: 58-64.

95. Casperson, C. J., K.E. Powell, G.M. Christenson. Physical activity, exercise, and physical fitness. *Public Health Rep*. 100 (1985): 125-131.

96. American College of Sports Medicine. The female athlete triad. (Position Stand). Med. *Sci. Sports and Exer*. 29.5 (1997), i-ix.

Appendix A
Suggested Reading

BOOKS

General Fitness and Health, Exercise Testing and Prescription

ACSM's Health/Fitness Facility Standards and Guidelines. 2nd ed. Eds. S. Tharrett and J. Peterson. Champaign: Human Kinetics Pub., 1997.

American College of Sports Medicine Guidelines for Exercise Testing and Prescription (6th ed.). Lippincott Williams & Wilkins, Baltimore, MD, 2000.

American College of Sports Medicine Resource Manual for Guidelines for Exercise Testing and Prescription (3rd ed.). Lippincott Williams & Wilkins, Baltimore, MD, 1998.

An Emerging Profession: The Fitness Practitioner. Eds. N. Sol and L. Gladwin. Sherman Oaks: AFAA, 1996.

Exercise, Fitness, and Health: International Proceedings and Consensus Statement. Eds. C. Bouchard, R.J. Shephard, and T. Stephens. Champaign: Human Kinetics Pub., 1994.

Exercise in Health and Disease. 2nd ed. M.L. Pollock and J.H.W.B. Wilmore. Philadelphia: Saunders Co., 1990.

Fitness: Theory & Practice. 2nd ed. Ed. Peg Jordan. Sherman Oaks: AFAA (and Stoughton: Reebok University Press), 1995.

Health Fitness Instructor's Handbook. 2nd ed. E.T. Howley and B.D. Franks. Champaign: Human Kinetics Pub., 1992.

Personal Trainer Manual, The Resource for Fitness Instructors. Ed. M. Sudy. San Diego: American Council on Exercise, 1991.

Y's Way to Physical Fitness: Complete Guide to Fitness Testing and Instruction. 3rd ed. L.A. Golding, C.R. Meyers, and W.E. Sinning. Champaign: Human Kinetics Pub., 1989.

Fitness Assessment

Advanced Fitness Assessment and Exercise Prescription. 2nd ed. V.H. Heyward. Champaign: Human Kinetics Pub., 1991.

Anthropometric Standardization Reference Manual. Eds. T.G. Lohman, A.F. Roche, and R. Martorell, R. Champaign: Human Kinetics Pub., 1991.

Applied Body Composition Assessment. V.H. Heyward and L.M. Stolarezy. Champaign: Human Kinetics Pub., 1996.

Physiological Assessment of Human Fitness. Eds. P.J. Maud and C. Foster. Champaign: Human Kinetics Pub., 1995.

Wellness and Health

Pathways to Wellness. S.R. Dickman. Champaign: Human Kinetics Pub., 1988.

The University of California, Berkeley Wellness Encyclopedia. Editors of the University of California, Berkeley Wellness Letter. Boston: Houghton Mifflin Co., 1991.

Wellness: Small Changes You Can Use to Make a Big Difference. R.S. Ryan and S.W. Travis. Berkeley: Ten Speed Press, 1991.

Physiology

Exercise Physiology. 3rd ed. W.D. McArdle, F.I. Katch, and V.L. Katch. Philadelphia: Lea & Febiger, 1990.

METCALC Software (Metabolic Calculations in Exercise and Fitness). N.K. Ng. Champaign: Human Kinetics Pub., 1995.

Physiological Basis for Exercise and Sport. 5th ed. E.L. Fox, R.W. Bowers, and M.L. Foss. Madison: Brown Benchmark Pub., 1993.

Physiology of Sport And Exercise. J.H. Wilmore and D.L. Costill. Champaign: Human Kinetics Pub., 1994.

Practical Math for Health Fitness Professionals. D.K. Flood. Champaign: Human Kinetics Pub., 1996.

Textbook of Medical Physiology. 7th ed. A.C.W.B. Guyton. Philadelphia: Saunders Co., 1986.

Resistance Training

Designing Resistance Training Programs. S.J. Fleck and W.J. Kraemer. Champaign: Human Kinetics Pub., 1987.

Essentials of Strength Training and Conditioning. Ed. T.R. Baechle. Champaign: Human Kinetics Pub., 1994.

Explosive Power and Strength. D.A. Chu. Champaign: Human Kinetics Pub., 1996.

Strength Fitness. 3rd ed. W. Westcott. Dubuque: Wm. C. Brown Pub., 1991.

Strength Training for Young Athletes. W.J. Kraemer and S.J. Fleck. Champaign: Human Kinetics Pub., 1993.

Touch Training for Strength. B. Rothenberg and O. Rothenberg. Champaign: Human Kinetics Pub., 1995.

Weight Training Instruction: Steps to Success. T.R. Baechle and B.R. Groves. Champaign: Human Kinetics Pub., 1994.

Flexibility Training

Facilitated Stretching: PNF Stretching Made Easy. R.E. McAtee. Champaign: Human Kinetics Pub., 1993.

Science of Stretching. 2nd ed. M.J. Alter. Champaign: Human Kinetics Pub., 1996.

Sport Stretch. M.J. Alter. Champaign: Human Kinetics Pub., 1990.

Stretching. B. Anderson. Bolinas: Shelter Publications, 1980.

Kinesiology and Functional Anatomy

Anatomy of Movement. B. Calais-Germain. Seattle: Eastland Press, Inc., 1993.

Brunnstrom's Clinical Kinesiology. 4th ed. L.D. Lehmkuhl and L.K. Smith. Philadelphia: F.A. Davis Co., 1983.

Joint Structure and Function, A Comprehensive Analysis. 2nd ed. C.C. Norkin and P.K. Levangie. Philadelphia: F.A. Davis Co., 1992.

Kinesiology. 7th ed. K. Luttgens and K.F.W.B. Wells. Philadelphia: Saunders Pub., 1982.

Kinesiology and Applied Anatomy. 7th ed. P.J. Rasch. Baltimore: Williams & Wilkins, 1989.

Manual of Structural Kinesiology. 12th ed. C.W. Thompson and R.T. Floyd. St. Louis: Mosby Year Book, Inc., 1994.

Neuromechanical Basis of Kinesiology. 2nd ed. R.M. Enoka. Champaign: Human Kinetics Pub., 1994.

Special Populations

ACSM's Exercise Management for Persons with Chronic Diseases and Disabilities. Ed. J.L. Durstine, Ph.D. Champaign: Human Kinetics Pub., 1997.

Arthritis: Your Complete Exercise Guide. N.F. Gordon. Champaign: Human Kinetics Pub., 1993.

Biomarkers: The 10 Keys to Prolonging Vitality. W. Evans and I.H. Rosenberg. New York: Simon and Schuster, 1991.

Diabetes: Your Complete Exercise Guide. N.F. Gordon. Champaign: Human Kinetics Pub., 1993.

Essential Exercises for the Childbearing Years. 3rd ed. E. Noble. Boston: Houghton Mifflin Co., 1988.

Exercise in Pregnancy. 2nd ed. Eds. R. Artal Mittelmark, R.A. Wiswell, and B.L. Drinkwater. Baltimore: Williams & Wilkins, 1991.

Exercise for Prevention and Treatment of Illness. L. Goldberg and D.L. Elliot. Philadelphia: P.A. Davis Co., 1994.

Exercise Programming for Older Adults. Ed. J. Clark. The Haworth Press, Inc. 1996.

Exercise Testing and Exercise Prescription for Special Cases. 2nd ed. J.S. Skinner. Baltimore: Williams & Wilkins, 1993.

Fit for Two: The Official YMCA Prenatal Exercise Guide. The YMCA of the USA with T.W. Hanlon. Champaign: Human Kinetics Pub., 1994.

Full Life Fitness. J. Clark. Champaign: Human Kinetics Pub., 1992.

Shaping Up for a Healthy Pregnancy: Instructor Guide. B.B. Holstein. Champaign: Human Kinetics Pub., 1988.

Stroke: Your Complete Exercise Guide. N.F. Gordon. Champaign: Human Kinetics Pub., 1993.

Understand Your Backache. R. Cailliet. Philadelphia: F.A. Davis Co., 1987.

Water Fitness During your Pregnancy. J. Katz. Champaign: Human Kinetics Pub., 1995.

YMCA Healthy Back Book. YMCA of the USA with P. Sammann. Champaign: Human Kinetics Pub., 1994.

Nutrition

Eating on the Run. 2nd ed. E. Tribole. Champaign: Human Kinetics Pub., 1992.

Helping Athletes with Eating Disorders. R.A. Thompson. R. Trattner Sherman. Champaign: Human Kinetics Pub., 1993.

LEARN Program for Weight Control. K.D. Brownell. 1994. Available through LEARN Education Center, Dallas, TX. (800) 736-7323.

Nancy Clark's Sports Nutrition Guidebook. N. Clark. Champaign: Human Kinetics Pub., 1990.

Nutrition and Exercise in Obesity Management. Eds. J. Storlie and H.A. Jordan. Champaign: Human Kinetics Pub., 1984.

Nutrition in Health. 8th ed. B. Shils. Baltimore: Williams & Wilkins, 1993.

The Balancing Act: Nutrition and Weight Guide. G. Kostas. Dallas: Cooper's Institute of Aerobics Research, 1993.

Understanding and Managing Cholesterol: A Guide for Wellness Professionals. K.P. Byrne. Champaign: Human Kinetics Pub., 1991.

Behavior Modification and Psychology

Advances in Exercise Adherence. Ed. R. Dishman. Champaign: Human Kinetics Pub., 1994.

Fitness Motivation: Preventing Participant Dropout. W.J. Rejeski and E.A. Kenney. Champaign: Human Kinetics Pub., 1988.

Psychology for Health Fitness Professionals. J. Gavin and N. Gavin. Champaign: Human Kinetics Pub., 1995.

Business

The Business of Personal Training. Ed. S.O. Roberts. Champaign: Human Kinetics Pub., 1996.

Legal Issues

An Emerging Profession: The Fitness Practitioner. Eds. N. Sol and L. Gladwin. Sherman Oaks: AFAA, 1996.

Legal Aspects of Personal Training. B.E. Koeberle. Canton: Professional Reports Corp., 1990.

Legal Aspects of Preventive, Rehabilitative and Recreational Exercise Programs. 3rd ed. D.L. Herbert and W.G. Herbert. Canton: PRC Publishing, Inc., 1993.

General Reference

Stedman's Medical Dictionary. 26th ed. Baltimore: Williams & Wilkins, 1995.

Physicians' Desk Reference. 50th ed. Montvale: Medical Economics Data Pub., 1996.

Journals and Magazines

ACSM's Health & Fitness Journal
Williams & Wilkins
P.O. Box 23291
Baltimore, MD 21203-9990

American Fitness
15250 Ventura Blvd. Ste. 200
Sherman Oaks, CA 91403

American Journal of Health Promotion
1812 S. Rochester Rd. Ste. 200
Rochester Hills, MI 48307

Exercise Standards and Malpractice Reporter
4418 Belden Village St., NW
Canton, OH 44718

Fitness Management
3923 W. Sixth St.
Los Angeles, CA 90020

IDEA Today and *IDEA Personal Trainer*
6190 Cornerstone Court East, Ste. 204
San Diego, CA 92121

Journal of Dance Medicine & Science
J. Michael Ryan Publishing, Inc.
24 Crescent Drive North
Andover, New Jersey 07821-4000

Medicine & Science in Sports & Exercise (ACSM)
401 W. Michigan St.
Indianapolis, IN 46202

Penn State Sports Medicine Newsletter
P.O. Box 6568
Syracuse, NY 13217

Sport Medicine Digest
Raven Press, Dept. 1B
1185 Ave. of the Americas
New York, NY 10036

Strength and Conditioning (NSCA)
P.O. Box 81410
920 O St.
Lincoln, NE 68508

The Physician and Sportsmedicine
4530 W. 77th St.
Minneapolis, MN 55435

Tufts Diet and Nutrition Letter
53 Park Place
New York, NY 10007

UC Berkeley Wellness Letter
P.O. Box 420148
Palm Coast, FL 32142

Appendix B

Personal Fitness Trainer Forms and Questionnaires

Legal Forms

The following legal forms have been reproduced with permission from *Legal Aspects of Personal Fitness Training* by Brian E. Koeberle, J.D., 1990, published by PRC Publishing, Inc., 4418 Belden Village Street, N.W., Canton, OH 44718-2516. All rights reserved. From *Legal Aspects of Preventive, Rehabilitative and Recreational Exercise Programs*, Third Edition, by David L. Herbert, J.D. and William G. Herbert, Ph.D., published by PRC Publishing, Inc., 1993, 4418 Belden Village Street, NW, Canton, OH 44718-2516. All rights reserved.

Release of Information Form

TO WHOM IT MAY CONCERN:

Please furnish to _____ (hereinafter "Facility") and/or any or all of its personnel, information, copies of any and all hospital and medical records or reports of any sort, charts, notes, x-rays, lab reports and prescription information, including the right to inspect and copy such records. Facility is to be furnished any and all other information without limitation pertaining to any confinement, examination, treatment or condition of myself, including medical, dental, psychological or other treatment, examinations, or counseling for any condition, medical, dental or psychological.

This AUTHORIZATION shall be considered as continuing and you may rely upon it in all respects unless you have previously been advised by me in writing to the contrary. It is expressly understood by the undersigned and you are hereby authorized to accept a copy or photocopy of this medical authorization with the same validity as though an original had been presented to you.

Dated this _____ day of_____, 20 _____.

Signature: _____

Name: _____

Address: _____

_____

Phone: _____

Physician Referral Form for Candidate to Enter Cardiac Therapy or Adult Fitness Programs

Please complete the following:

Name of Patient: _____ Date: _____

Address: _____ Age: _____

Phone:_____ Sex:_____ SS#: _____

Date of Last Completed Examination: ___/___/___

Cardiovascular Disease Diagnosis:

      Post-MI; Date of Hospitalization   ___/___/___

      Post-CABG; Date of Surgery   ___/___/___

      Angina; Date of Diagnosis   ___/___/___

      Hypertension; Date of Diagnosis   ___/___/___

      Rhythm Abnormality; Date of Diagnosis   ___/___/___

      Claudication; Date of Diagnosis   ___/___/___

      Other; Date of Diagnosis   ___/___/___

CAD Risk Factors:

Hypercholesterolemia	Hyperglycemia or Diabetes
Abnormal Lipoprotein Level	Obesity
Smoking	Sedentary Lifestyle
Family History of Early CAD	Tension/Stress

Current Medications

Special Considerations	Medication	Dose	Frequency
Syncope	_____	_____	_____
Musculoskeletal Disorders	_____	_____	_____
Asthma	_____	_____	_____
Other	_____	_____	_____

Please fill in/enclose following information, if it is already available in patient's records:

A. 12-lead EKG (optional for those under 35 years of age; desired for those over 35)

B. Blood pressure: Systolic/Diastolic (arm) _____/_____ (   )

C. Serum Cholesterol_____mg/dl

D. Triglycerides_____mg/dl

E. Previous graded exercise test results (if available)

I have examined the above applicant and as his/her personal physician approve participation in:

_____ Hospital Cardiac Outpatient Program (continuous supervision and ECG monitoring)

_____ Community Cardiac Outpatient Program (continuous supervision, intermittent ECG monitoring)

_____ Adult Fitness Program (intermittent supervision, no ECG monitoring)

Any special exercise limitations are listed below:

_____

_____

Signed: _____

Phone: (_____) _____

Physician

Name of Physician: (Print) _____

Address: _____

Return to: (Program Office) _____

_____

_____

Informed Consent for Exercise Testing
of Apparently Healthy Adults
(without known heart disease)

Name: _____

1. Purpose and Explanation of Test

I hereby consent to voluntarily engage in an exercise test to determine my circulatory and respiratory fitness. I also consent to the taking of samples of my exhaled air during exercise to properly measure my oxygen consumption. I also consent, if necessary, to have a small blood sample drawn by needle from my arm for blood chemistry analysis and to the performance of lung function and body fat (skinfold pinch) tests. It is my understanding that the information obtained will help me evaluate future physical activities and sports activities in which I may engage.

Before I undergo the test, I certify to the program that I am in good health and have had a physical examination conducted by a licensed medical physician within the last _____ months. Further, I hereby represent and inform the program that I have completed the pre-test history interview presented to me by the program staff and have provided correct responses to the questions as indicated on the history form or as supplied to the interviewer. It is my understanding that I will be interviewed by a physician or other person prior to my undergoing the test who will in the course of interviewing me determine if there are any reasons which would make it undesirable or unsafe for me to take the test. Consequently, I understand that it is important that I provide complete and accurate responses to the interviewer and recognize that my failure to do so could lead to possible unnecessary injury to myself during the test.

The test which I will undergo will be performed on a motor driven treadmill or bicycle ergometer with the amount of effort gradually increasing. As I understand it, this increase in effort will continue until I feel and verbally report to the operator any symptoms such as fatigue, shortness of breath or chest discomfort which may appear. It is my understanding and I have been clearly advised that it is my right to request that a test be stopped at any point if I feel unusual discomfort or fatigue. I have been advised that I should immediately, upon experiencing any such symptoms or if I so choose, inform the operator that I wish to stop the test at that or any other point. My wishes in this regard shall be absolutely carried out.

It is further my understanding that prior to beginning the test, I will be connected by electrodes and cables to an electrocardiographic recorder which will enable the program personnel to monitor my cardiac (heart) activity. During the test itself, it is my understanding that a trained observer will monitor my responses continuously and take frequent readings of blood pressure, the electrocardiogram, and my expressed feelings of effort. I realize that a true determination of my exercise capacity depends on progressing the test to the point of my fatigue.

Once the test has been completed, but before I am released from the test area, I will be given special instructions about showering and recognition of certain symptoms which may appear within the first 24 hours after the test. I agree to follow these instructions and promptly contact the program personnel or medical providers if such symptoms develop.

2. Risks

It is my understanding and I have been informed that there exists the possibility of adverse changes during the actual test. I have been informed that these changes could include abnormal blood pressure, fainting, disorders of heart rhythm, stroke and very rare instances of heart attack or even death. Every effort, I have been told, will be made to minimize these occurrences by preliminary examination and by precautions and observations taken during the test. I have also been informed that emergency equipment and personnel are readily available to deal with these unusual situations should they occur. I understand that there is a risk of injury, heart attack, stroke or even death as a result of my performance of this test, but knowing those risks, it is my desire to proceed to take the test as herein indicated.

3. Benefits to be Expected and Alternatives Available to the Exercise Testing Procedure

The results of this test may or may not benefit me. Potential benefits relate mainly to my personal motives for taking the test, i.e., knowing my exercise capacity in relation to the general population, understanding my fitness for certain sports and recreational activities, planning my physical conditioning program or evaluating the effects of my recent physical activity habits. Although my fitness might also be evaluated by alternative means, e.g., a bench step test or an outdoor running test, such tests do not provide as accurate a fitness assessment as the treadmill or bike test nor do those options allow equally effective monitoring of my responses.

4. Confidentiality and Use of Information

I have been informed that the information which is obtained in this exercise test will be treated as privileged and confidential and will consequently not be released or revealed to any person without my express written consent. I do, however, agree to the use of any information for research or statistical purposes so long as same does not provide facts which could lead to the identification of my person. Any other information obtained, however, will be used only by the program staff to evaluate my exercise status or needs.

5. Inquiries and Freedom of Consent

I have been given an opportunity to ask questions as to the procedure. Generally these requests, which have been noted by the testing staff, and their responses are as follows:

_____

_____

I further understand that there are also other remote risks that may be associated with this procedure. Despite the fact that a complete accounting of all remote risks is not entirely possible, I am satisfied with the review of these risks which was provided to me and it is still my desire to proceed with the test.

I acknowledge that I have read this document in its entirety or that it has been read to me if I have been unable to read same.

I consent to the rendition of all services and procedures as explained herein by all program personnel and to the provision of emergency care response and CPR if necessary.

Date _____   _____
                                                  Participant's Signature

_____
    Witness' Signature

_____
  Test Supervisor's Signature

Alternative Form for
Informed Consent for Exercise Testing
Procedures of Apparently Healthy Adults

Name: _____

1. Purpose and Explanation of Test

It is my understanding that I will undergo a test to be performed on a motor driven treadmill or bicycle ergometer with the amount of effort gradually increasing. As I understand it, this increase in effort will continue until I feel and verbally report to the operator any symptoms such as fatigue, shortness of breath or chest discomfort which may appear or until the test is completed or otherwise terminated. It is my understanding and I have been clearly advised that it is my right to request that a test be stopped at any point if I feel unusual discomfort or fatigue. I have been advised that I should immediately, upon experiencing any such symptoms or if I so choose, inform the operator that I wish to stop the test at that or any other point. My stated wishes in this regard shall be carried out. **IF CORRECT AND YOU AGREE AND UNDERSTAND, INITIAL HERE _____.**

It is further my understanding that prior to beginning the test, I will be connected by electrodes and cables to an electrocardiographic recorder which will enable the program personnel to monitor my cardiac (heart) activity. During the test itself, it is my understanding that a trained observer will monitor my responses continuously and take frequent readings of blood pressure, the electrocardiogram and my expressed feelings of effort. I realize that a true determination of my exercise capacity depends on progressing the test to a point of my fatigue. Once the test has been completed, but before I am released from the test area, I will be given special instructions about showering and recognition of certain symptoms which may appear within the first 24 hours after the test. I agree to follow these instructions and promptly contact the program personnel or medical providers if such symptoms develop. **IF CORRECT AND YOU AGREE AND UNDERSTAND, INITIAL HERE _____.**

Before I undergo the test, I certify to the program that I am in good health and have had a physical examination conducted by a licensed medical physician within the last _____ months. Further, I hereby represent and inform the program that I have accurately completed the pre-test history interview presented to me by the program staff and have provided correct responses to the questions as indicated on the history form or as supplied to the interviewer. It is my understanding that I will be interviewed by a physician or other person prior to my undergoing the test who will, in the course of interviewing me, determine if there are any reasons which would make it undesirable or unsafe for me to take the test. Consequently, I understand that it is important that I provide complete and accurate responses to the interviewer and recognize that my failure to do so could lead to possible unnecessary injury to myself during the test. **IF CORRECT AND YOU AGREE, INITIAL HERE** _____.

2. Risks

It is my understanding, and I have been informed, that there exists the possibility of adverse changes during the actual test. I have been informed that these changes could include abnormal blood pressure, fainting, disorders of heart rhythm, stroke and very rare instances of heart attack or even death. I have also been informed that aside from the foregoing other risks exist. These risks include, but are not necessarily limited to the possibility of stroke, or other cerebrovascular or cardiovascular incident or occurrence, mental, physiological, motor, visual or hearing injuries, deficiencies, difficulties or disturbances, partial or total paralysis, slips, falls, or other unintended loss of balance or bodily movement related to the exercise treadmill (or bicycle ergometer) which may cause muscular, neurological, orthopedic or other bodily injury as well as a variety of other possible occurrences, any one of which could conceivably, however remotely, cause bodily injury, impairment, disability or death. Any procedure such as this one carries with it some risk however unlikely or remote. THERE ARE ALSO OTHER RISKS OF INJURY, IMPAIRMENT, DISABILITY, DISFIGUREMENT, AND EVEN DEATH. I ACKNOWLEDGE AND AGREE TO ASSUME ALL RISKS. **IF YOU UNDERSTAND AND AGREE, INITIAL HERE** _____.

Every effort, I have been told, will be made to minimize these occurrences by preliminary examination and by precautions and observations taken during the test. I have also been informed that emergency equipment and personnel are readily available to deal with these unusual situations should they occur.

Knowing and understanding all risks, it is my desire to proceed to take the test as herein described. **IF CORRECT AND YOU AGREE AND UNDERSTAND, INITIAL HERE** _____.

3. Benefits to be Expected and Alternatives Available to the Exercise Testing Procedure

I understand and have been told that the results of this test may or may not benefit me. Potential benefits relate mainly to my personal motives for taking the test, i.e., knowing my exercise capacity in relation to the general population, understanding my fitness for certain sports and recreational activities, planning my physical conditioning program or evaluating the effects of my recent physical activity habits. Although my fitness might also be evaluated by alternative means, e.g., a bench step test or an outdoor running test, such tests do not provide as accurate a fitness assessment as the treadmill or bike test nor do those options allow equally effective monitoring of my responses. **IF YOU UNDERSTAND, INITIAL HERE** _____.

4. Consent

I hereby consent to voluntarily engage in an exercise test to determine my circulatory and respiratory fitness. I also consent to the taking of samples of my exhaled air during exercise to properly measure my oxygen consumption. I also consent, if necessary, to have a small blood sample drawn by needle from my arm for blood chemistry analysis and to the performance of lung function and body fat (skinfold pinch) tests. It is my understanding that the information obtained will help me evaluate future physical fitness and sports activities in which I may engage. **IF CORRECT AND YOU AGREE, INITIAL HERE** _____.

5. Confidentiality and Use of Information

I have been informed that the information which is obtained in this exercise test will be treated as privileged and confidential and will consequently not be released or revealed to any person without my express written consent. I do, however, agree to the use of any information for research or statistical purposes, so long as same does not provide facts which could lead to the identification of my person. Any other information obtained, however, will be used only by the program staff to evaluate my exercise status or needs. **IF YOU AGREE, INITIAL HERE** _____.

6. Inquiries and Freedom of Consent

I have been given an opportunity to ask questions as to the procedures. Generally these requests, which have been noted by the testing staff, and their responses are as follows:

_____

_____

IF THIS NOTATION IS COMPLETE AND CORRECT, INITIAL HERE _____.

I acknowledge that I have read this document in its entirety or that it has been read to me if I have been unable to read same.

I consent to the rendition of all services and procedures as explained herein by all program personnel and to the provision of emergency care response and CPR if necessary.

I consent to the rendition of all services and procedures as explained herein by all program personnel and to the provision of emergency care response and CPR if necessary.

Date _____

_____
Witness' Signature

_____
Participant's Signature

_____
Witness' Signature

_____
Spouse's Consent

_____
Test Supervisor's Signature

Informed Consent for Participation in an Exercise Program for Apparently Healthy Adults
(without known or suspected heart disease)

Name: _____

1. Purpose and Explanation of Procedure

I hereby consent to voluntarily engage in an acceptable plan of exercise conditioning. I also give consent to be placed in program activities which are recommended to me for improvement of my general health and well-being. These may include dietary counseling, stress reduction, and health education activities. The levels of exercise which I will perform will be based upon my cardiorespiratory (heart and lungs) fitness as determined through my recent laboratory graded exercise evaluation. I will be given exact instructions regarding the amount and kind of exercise I should do. I agree to participate three times per week in the formal program sessions. Professionally trained personnel will provide leadership to direct my activities, monitor my performance, and otherwise evaluate my effort. Depending upon my health status, I may or may not be required to have my blood pressure and heart rate evaluated during these sessions to regulate my exercise within desired limits. I understand that I am expected to attend every session and to follow staff instructions with regard to exercise, diet, stress management, and smoking cessation. If I am taking prescribed medications, I have already so informed the program staff and further agree to so inform them promptly of any changes which my doctor or I have made with regard to use of these. I will be given the opportunity for periodic assessment with laboratory evaluations at 6 months after the start of my program. Should I remain in the program thereafter, additional evaluations will generally be given at 12 month intervals. The program may change the foregoing schedule of evaluations, if this is considered desirable for health reasons.

I have been informed that during my participation in exercise, I will be asked to complete the physical activities unless symptoms such as fatigue, shortness of breath, chest discomfort or similar occurrences appear. At that point, I have been advised it is my complete right to decrease or stop exercise and that it is my obligation to inform the program personnel of my symptoms. I hereby state that I have been so advised and agree to inform the program personnel of my symptoms, should any develop.

I understand that during the performance of exercise, a trained observer will periodically monitor my performance and, perhaps measure my pulse, blood pressure or assess my feelings of effort for the purposes of monitoring my progress.

I also understand that the observer may reduce or stop my exercise program, when any of these findings so indicate that this should be done for my safety and benefit.

2. Risks

It is my understanding, and I have been so informed, that there exists the remote possibility during exercise of adverse changes, including abnormal blood pressure, fainting, disorders of heart rhythm, and very rare instances of heart attack, stroke or even death, as well as other risks of injury or impairment, due to my participation in activity. Every effort, I have been told, will be made to minimize these occurrences by proper staff assessment of my condition before each exercise session, staff supervision during exercise and by my own careful control of exercise efforts. I have also been informed that emergency equipment and personnel are readily available to deal with unusual situations should these occur. I understand that there is a risk of injury, heart attack or even death as a result of my exercise, but knowing those risks, it is my desire to participate as herein indicated.

3. Benefits to be Expected and Alternatives Available to Exercise

I understand that this program may or may not benefit my physical fitness or general health. I recognize that involvement in the exercise sessions will allow me to learn proper ways to perform conditioning exercises, use fitness equipment, and regulate physical effort. These experiences should benefit me by indicating how my physical limitations may affect my ability to perform various physical activities. I further understand that if I closely follow the program instructions, that I will likely improve my exercise capacity after a period of 3-6 months.

4. Confidentiality and Use of Information

I have been informed that the information which is obtained in this exercise program will be treated as privileged and confidential and will consequently not be released or revealed to any person without my express written consent. I do, however, agree to the use of any information which is not personally identifiable with me for research and statistical purposes so long as same does not identify my person or provide facts which could lead to my identification. Any other information obtained, however, will be used only by the program staff in the course of prescribing exercise for me and evaluating my progress in the program.

5. Inquiries and Freedom of Consent

I have been given an opportunity to ask certain questions as to the procedures of this program. Generally these requests, which have been noted by the interviewing staff member, and his/her responses are as follows:

_____

_____

_____

I further understand that there are also other remote risks that may be associated with this program. Despite the fact that a complete accounting of all these remote risks is not entirely possible, I am satisfied with the review of these risks which was provided to me and it is still my desire to participate.

I acknowledge that I have read this document in its entirety or that it has been read to me if I have been unable to read same.

I consent to the rendition of all services and procedures as explained herein by all program personnel and to the provision of emergency care response and CPR if necessary.

Date _____   _____
                                                                    Participant's Signature

_____
        Witness' Signature

_____
        Test Supervisor's Signature

Agreement and Release of Liability

1. In consideration of being allowed to participate in the activities and programs of
    _____ and to use its facilities, equipment and machinery, in
    addition to the payment of any fee or charge, I do hereby waive, release and
    forever discharge _____ and its directors, officers,
    agents, employees, representatives, successors and assigns, administrators,
    executors, and all others from any and all responsibilities or liability from
    injuries or damages resulting from my participation in any activities or my use
    of equipment or machinery in the above mentioned activities. I do also hereby
    release all of those mentioned and any others acting upon their behalf from any
    responsibility or liability for any injury or damage to myself, including those
    caused by the negligent act or omission of any of those mentioned or others
    acting on their behalf or in any way arising out of or connected with my
    participation in any activities of _____ or
    the use of any equipment at _____
    _____.
    IF YOU UNDERSTAND AND AGREE, PLEASE INITIAL_____.

2. I understand and am aware that strength, flexibility and aerobic exercise,
    including the use of equipment, is a potentially hazardous activity. I also
    understand that fitness activities involve the risk of injury and even death, and
    that I am voluntarily participating in these activities and using equipment and
    machinery with knowledge of the dangers involved. I hereby agree to expressly
    assume and accept any and all risks of injury or death.
    IF YOU UNDERSTAND AND AGREE, PLEASE INITIAL_____.

3. I do hereby further declare myself to be physically sound and suffering from no
    condition, impairment, disease, infirmity or other illness that would prevent my
    participation or use of equipment or machinery except as hereinafter stated. I do
    hereby acknowledge that I have been informed of the need for a physician's
    approval for my participation in an exercise/fitness activity or in the use of
    exercise equipment and machinery. I also acknowledge that it has been
    recommended that I have a yearly or more frequent physical examination and
    consultation with my physician as to physical activity, exercise and use of
    exercise and training equipment so that I might have his recommendations
    concerning these fitness activities and equipment use. I acknowledge that I have
    either had a physical examination and have been given my physician's
    permission to participate, or that I have decided to participate in activity and use

of equipment and machinery without the approval of my physician and do hereby assume all responsibility for my participation and activities, and utilization of equipment and machinery in my activities.

IF YOU UNDERSTAND AND AGREE, PLEASE INITIAL_____.

Date _____   _____

                                                                      Signature

Alternative Form—Express Assumption of Risk/Prospective Waiver of Liability and Release Agreement

I, the undersigned, hereby expressly and affirmatively state that I wish to participate in fitness assessments, activities and programs, and in the use of exercise equipment at various sites, including home, club or worksite, that may be provided or recommended by (_____)(hereinafter "Facility"). I realize that my participation in these activities or in the use of equipment involves various risks of injury including, but not limited to (list) _____

_____

_____

and even the possibility of death. I also recognize that there are many other risks of injury, including serious disabling injuries, that may arise due to my participation in these activities or in the use of equipment and that such risks, including remote ones, have been reviewed with me. I also understand that under some circumstances I may choose to engage in activity in a non-supervised setting under circumstances where there is no one to respond to any emergency that may arise as a result of my participation or use of equipment on an individual basis, in an unsupervised setting. Despite the fact that I have been duly cautioned as to such unsupervised and unattended activity or equipment use, and despite the fact that I have been advised against such activity and equipment use in an unsupervised and unattended setting, I, knowing the material risks and appreciating, knowing and reasonably anticipating that other injuries and even death are a possibility as a result of my participation in fitness assessments, activities or programs, or in the use of equipment in supervised/attended and unsupervised/unattended settings (within which settings I acknowledge that the risks of injury or death may be greater than in other settings), I hereby expressly assume all of the delineated risks of injury, all other possible risks of injury and even the risk of death which could occur by reason of my participation in any of the assessments, activities or programs, or in the use of equipment in any or all settings. **IF YOU UNDERSTAND AND AGREE, PLEASE INITIAL_____.**

I have had an opportunity to ask questions regarding my participation in various activities and in the use of exercise equipment. Any questions I have asked have been answered to my complete satisfaction. I subjectively understand the risks of my participation in various activities or in the use of equipment and knowing and appreciating these risks, I voluntarily choose to participate, assuming all risks of injury and death which may arise due to my participation. **IF YOU UNDERSTAND AND AGREE, PLEASE INITIAL_____.**

I further acknowledge that my participation in the activities and use of equipment is completely voluntary and that it is my choice to participate and/or reuse equipment or not to participate as I see fit. **IF YOU UNDERSTAND AND AGREE, PLEASE INITIAL_____.**

In consideration of being allowed to participate in the activities and programs provided through Facility and/or in the use of its facilities and equipment, I do hereby waive, release and forever discharge Facility, and all of its directors, officers, agents, employees, representatives, successors and assigns, and all others from any and all responsibility or liability for injuries or damages resulting from my participation in any activities at Facility or elsewhere. I do also hereby release all of those mentioned and any others acting on their behalf from any responsibility or liability for any injury or damage to myself, including those caused by the negligent act or omission of any of those mentioned or others acting on their behalf or in any way arising out of or connected with my participation in any of the contemplated activities or in the use of equipment through Facility or otherwise. **IF YOU UNDERSTAND AND AGREE, PLEASE INITIAL_____.**

I understand and am aware that strength, flexibility and aerobic exercise, including the use of equipment, are potentially hazardous activities. I also understand that fitness activities involve a risk of injury and even death and that I am voluntarily participating in these activities and using equipment with knowledge of the dangers involved. **IF YOU UNDERSTAND AND AGREE, PLEASE INITIAL _____.**

I do further declare myself to be physically sound and suffering from no condition, impairment, disease, infirmity or other illness that would prevent my participation in any of the activities and programs provided through Facility or in the use of equipment and machinery except as hereinafter stated: _____ _____. I do hereby acknowledge that I have been informed of the need or desirability for a physician's approval for my participation in exercise/fitness activity or in the use of exercise equipment. I also acknowledge that it has been recommended that I have a yearly or more frequent physical examination and consultation with my physician as to physical activities and exercise, and as to the use of exercise equipment, so that I might have recommendations concerning these physical activities and equipment use. I acknowledge that I have either had a physical examination and have been given my physician's permission to participate or that I have decided to participate in activity and/or use of equipment without the approval of my physician and do hereby assume all responsibility for my participation and activities or in the utilization of equipment without that approval. **IF YOU UNDERSTAND AND AGREE, PLEASE INITIAL _____.**

I, the undersigned spouse of the participant, do hereby further acknowledge that my spouse (participant) wishes to engage in certain activities and programs provided by

Facility including the use of various facilities and equipment. In consideration of my spouse's (participant's) voluntary decision to engage in such activities, and in consideration of the provision of such activities and equipment to spouse by Facility, I, the undersigned, do hereby waive, release and forever discharge Facility and its directors, officers, agents, employees, representatives, successors and assigns, and all others from any and all responsibility or liability for any injuries or damages resulting from my spouse's participation in any activities or in my spouse's use of equipment as a result of participation in any such activities or otherwise arising out of that participation. I do further release all of those mentioned above and any others acting on their behalf from any responsibility or liability for any injury to, or even death of, my spouse, including those caused by the negligent act or omission of any of those mentioned or others acting upon their behalf or in any way arising out of or connected with my spouse's participation in any of the activities provided by Facility or in the use of any equipment at any location. I specifically acknowledge that my execution of this prospective Waiver and Release relinquishes any cause of action that I may have either directly through my spouse or independently by way of a loss of consortium or other type of action of any kind or nature whatsoever, and I do hereby further agree to my spouse's participation in the activities as above mentioned and in the use of any equipment at any location. **IF SPOUSE UNDERSTANDS AND AGREES, SPOUSE TO INITIAL HERE _____.**

IN WITNESS WHEREOF, the participant and the participant's spouse, if any, have executed this Express Assumption of Risk/Prospective Waiver of Liability and Release Agreement this _____ day of_____, 20___, which shall be binding upon each of them and their respective heirs, executors, administrators and assigns. Each does hereby further agree to indemnify and hold Facility and all those identified or named herein absolutely harmless in the event that anyone claiming any cause of action as a result of any injury and/or death to participant or spouse attempts at any time to institute any claim or suit against the Facility arising out of any of the activities or programs herein or in the use of any equipment.

Signed in the presence of:

_____   _____
                                                            Participant

_____   _____
                                                       Participant's Spouse

_____

_____

Express Assumption of Risk
for Participation in Specified Activity

I, the undersigned, hereby expressly and affirmatively state that I wish to participate in _____. I realize that my participation in this activity involves risks of injury, including but not to limited to (list) _____ _____ and even the possibility of death. I also recognize that there are many other risks of injury, including serious disabling injuries, which may arise due to my participation in this activity and that it is not possible to specifically list each and every individual injury risk. However, knowing the material risks and appreciating, knowing and reasonably anticipating that other injuries and even death are a possibility, I hereby expressly assume all of the delineated risks of injury, all other possible risks of injury and even death which could occur by reason of my participation.

I have had an opportunity to ask questions. Any questions which I have asked have been answered to my complete satisfaction. I subjectively understand the risks of my participation in this activity, and knowing and appreciating these risks I voluntarily choose to participate, assuming all risks of injury or even death due to my participation.

_____   _____
Witness   Participant

Date _____

NOTES OF QUESTIONS AND ANSWERS

_____

_____

_____

This is as stated, a true and accurate record of what was asked and answered.

_____
Participant

FitMarkers

(The top five categories for determining health/fitness status)

Carefully read each question to the client. Fill in the appropriate space and check either yes or no. It is imperative that the client answer each question honestly.

State of Being

When was your last physical examination? (check appropriate box)

Within six months (acceptable) ❑

Within one year (acceptable) ❑

Has been over one year (unacceptable) ❑

What is your physician's name and phone number? (optional)

_____(_____)____

Sex: Male or Female? M ❑   F ❑

Age: Male >40 Female >50 Yes ❑ No ❑

What is your present height? _____

What is your present weight? _____

Family History

Has one or more close family member(s) been diagnosed
with coronary heart disease? Yes ❑ No ❑

Has one or more close family member(s) been diagnosed
with high blood pressure/hypertension? Yes ❑ No ❑

Has one or more close family member(s) suffered a stroke? Yes ❑ No ❑

Has one or more close family member(s) been diagnosed
with diabetes mellitus? Yes ❑ No ❑

General Health

How would you describe your health?
Good ❑   Average ❑   Poor ❑
Good with medical management and/or medications ❑

Is your resting blood pressure greater than or equal to 140/90 mm Hg
(140 systolic pressure/90 diastolic pressure)?   Yes ❑ No ❑ Unknown ❑

For the client's information:
• *Less than 140/90 mm Hg is a good indication that your risk for cardiovascular disease is low.*
• *140/90 mm Hg means you are borderline and should see a physician for verification and recommendation.*

• *Above 140/90 mm Hg means you are at risk for coronary heart disease (CHD) and need medical attention.*
• *If you are unsure of your resting blood pressure you should see a physician to determine if you fall within the healthy range.*

Is your blood serum cholesterol
level >200 mg/dL?   Yes ❑   No ❑   Unknown ❑
Has your physician determined
your cholesterol/HDL ratio?   Yes ❑   No ❑   Unknown ❑

For the client's information the tables below show guidelines in regard to cholesterol.

Cholesterol Levels and CHD Risk

	Total Cholesterol	LDL Cholesterol
Desirable	<200 mg/dL	<130 mg/dL
Borderline	200–239 mg/dL	130–159 mg/dL
High	>240 mg/dL	>160 mg/dL

Fasting Triglycerides

Age	Increased Risk
19–29	>140 mg/dL
30–39	>150 mg/dL
40–49	>160 mg/dL
>49	>190 mg/dL

CHD Risk Factors / Cholesterol/HDL Ratio

Ranking	Male	Female
$1/2$ of Average	3.4	3.3
Average (normal)	5.0	4.4
Twice Average (moderate)	9.6	7.0
Three Times Average (high)	13.4	11.0

(Data based on Framingham Study)
Note:
>Greater than
≥Greater than or equal to
<Less than
≤Less than or equal to

Have you been diagnosed with CHD?   Yes ❑   No ❑

Have you suffered a stroke?   Yes ❑   No ❑

Do you suffer from any stress-related symptoms?   Yes ❑   No ❑

    Extreme nervousness   Yes ❑   No ❑

    Problems sleeping   Yes ❑   No ❑

    Problems maintaining weight   Yes ❑   No ❑

    A consistently high resting heart rate   Yes ❑   No ❑

Have you experienced any of the following symptoms in the past month?

    Chest pains when physically inactive or
    when physically active   Yes ❑   No ❑

    Shortness of breath climbing a flight of stairs   Yes ❑   No ❑

    Dizziness when rising from bed or
    a chair or anytime throughout the day   Yes ❑   No ❑

    A loss of consciousness   Yes ❑   No ❑

    Have you been diagnosed with diabetes mellitus?   Yes ❑   No ❑

    If yes, Type I ❑ Type II ❑

Special Health Considerations

Have you had any surgeries within the past year?   Yes ❑   No ❑

If so, please state reason _____

_____

Do you have any of the following limiting physical conditions?

    Pregnancy   Yes ❑   No ❑

    Muscular dystrophy   Yes ❑   No ❑

    Nerve or sensory damage   Yes ❑   No ❑

    Multiple sclerosis   Yes ❑   No ❑

    Other _____

Do you suffer from any of the following limiting orthopedic conditions?

    Arthritis   Yes ❑   No ❑

    Bursitis   Yes ❑   No ❑

    Broken bones   Yes ❑   No ❑

    Stress fractures   Yes ❑   No ❑

    Prosthesis (hip, knee replacement, etc.)   Yes ❑   No ❑

    Other _____

Are you on any of the following medications?

Heart medications	Yes ❏	No ❏
Hypertensive medications	Yes ❏	No ❏
Asthma medications	Yes ❏	No ❏
Insulin injections	Yes ❏	No ❏
Water pills	Yes ❏	No ❏

Other _____

Environmental and Lifestyle Factors

Do you tend to eat meals high in dietary fat?	Yes ❏	No ❏
Are you sedentary (do not exercise at all)?	Yes ❏	No ❏
Do you exercise less than three to five times per week on a regular basis?	Yes ❏	No ❏

How would you describe your fitness ability?

Good ❏ Average ❏ Poor ❏

Do you sleep less than six hours per night?	Yes ❏	No ❏
Do you drink more than two glasses of alcohol per day?	Yes ❏	No ❏
Do you currently smoke cigarettes?	Yes ❏	No ❏
Were you a heavy smoker who recently quit?	Yes ❏	No ❏

If the client answers **yes** to one or more of the questions listed above, his/her FitMarkers status falls within the questionable range and, therefore, it is important for the client to consult with his/her physician and receive medical clearance before participating in any form of physical activity.

If the client has honestly answered **no** to each question, his/her FitMarkers status falls within the acceptable range and the client should be physically healthy enough to proceed with the following:

1. An exercise fitness test evaluating aerobic fitness, muscle strength and endurance, flexibility and body composition.

2. A **slow** progression into a regular exercise program (begin to exercise at a slow and relatively low intensity and then gradually build intensity).

When in doubt, always advise an individual to seek professional medical advice and screening.

Medical History Form

Name: _____ Date: _____

Telephone: _____

Date of Birth: _____ Age: _____ Height: _____ Weight: _____

In Case of Emergency Contact: _____ Relationship: _____

Address: _____ Phone: _____

Physician: _____ Specialty: _____

Address: _____ Phone: _____

Are you currently under a doctor's care?   Yes ❑   No ❑
  If yes, explain: _____

When was the last time you had a physical examination? _____

Have you ever had an exercise stress test: Yes ❑ No ❑ Don't know ❑

If yes, were the results: Normal ❑ Abnormal ❑

Do you take any medications on a regular basis?   Yes ❑   No ❑
  If yes, please list medications and reasons for taking: _____

_____

Have you been recently hospitalized?   Yes ❑   No ❑
  If yes, please explain: _____

_____

Do you smoke?   Yes ❑   No ❑
Are you pregnant?   Yes ❑   No ❑
Do you drink alcohol more than three times/week?   Yes ❑   No ❑
Is your stress level high?   Yes ❑   No ❑
Are you moderately active on most days of the week?   Yes ❑   No ❑

Do you have:
    High blood pressure?   Yes ❑   No ❑
    High cholesterol?   Yes ❑   No ❑
    Diabetes?   Yes ❑   No ❑

Have parents or siblings who, prior to age 55, had:
    A heart attack?   Yes ❑   No ❑
    A stroke?   Yes ❑   No ❑
    High blood pressure?   Yes ❑   No ❑
    High cholesterol?   Yes ❑   No ❑

Known heart disease?	Yes ❏ No ❏
Rheumatic heart disease?	Yes ❏ No ❏
A heart murmur?	Yes ❏ No ❏
Chest pain with exertion?	Yes ❏ No ❏
Irregular heart beat or palpitations?	Yes ❏ No ❏
Lightheadedness or do you faint?	Yes ❏ No ❏
Unusual shortness of breath?	Yes ❏ No ❏
Cramping pains in legs or feet?	Yes ❏ No ❏
Emphysema?	Yes ❏ No ❏
Other metabolic disorders (thyroid, kidney, etc.)?	Yes ❏ No ❏
Epilepsy?	Yes ❏ No ❏
Asthma?	Yes ❏ No ❏
Back pain: upper, middle, lower?	Yes ❏ No ❏
Other joint pain (explain on back of form)?	Yes ❏ No ❏
Muscle pain or an injury (explain on back of Form)?	Yes ❏ No ❏

To the best of my knowledge, the above information is true.

Signature _____

Date _____ Witness _____

Physician's Clearance Form

Please return this form to: _____

(Personal Trainer's name) _____

Address: _____

Phone: _____

Date: _____

Patient's name: _____ Age: _____

Date of last physical examination: _____

_____ This patient may participate fully in a physical activity program consisting of cardiovascular, strength, and flexibility training without limitation.

_____ This patient may participate in a physical activity program with the following limitations and/or recommendations: _____

_____

_____

Please include a brief description of any medical condition that might affect his/her physical activity program: _____

_____

If this patient is on any medication that may affect the heart rate or the blood pressure response to exercise (elevating or suppressing), please indicate:

I consider the above individual to be: _____ normal

_____ cardiac patient

_____ prone to coronary heart disease

_____ other (explain)

Please fill in the following information if available:

result of last GXT _____

blood pressure _____

glucose _____

total serum cholesterol _____

HDL-C _____ LDL-C _____

triglycerides _____

Physician's Signature _____ Date _____

Please Note: This record must be stamped with a physician's official stamp or be accompanied by a typed letter on a physician's letterhead, documenting that a medical evaluation has been performed on the named client. THE PHYSICIAN'S CLEARANCE FORM WILL NOT BE ACCEPTED WITHOUT SUCH PROPER VERIFICATION.

Exercise and Activity Quiz

Name: _____ Date: _____

How fit do you feel now? _____
(assign #1-5 with 1 being poor and 5 being excellent)

Exercise/activity habits:

In an average day, I climb _____ flights of stairs (~12 stairs/flight).

My job requires that I be on my feet and moving _____ hours a day
(example: waitress, industrial inspector, nurse). Count actual time
moving only.

My job requires that I be on my feet _____ hours a day, but I move around
very little (example: sales clerk).

In an average day I walk _____ miles (walking at least one mile at a time
without stopping).

I spend about _____ hours a week tending a garden or lawn.

I am a parent who assumes primary responsibility for a preschool child _____ .
— child and parent at home all day
— child spends half day in day care
— child spends full day in day care

My job is physically demanding (lifting, carrying, shoveling, climbing) for
_____ hours a day (consider only the time you are actually involved in
vigorous activity).

I perform household chores (laundry, cleaning, cooking) an average of _____
hours a week.

I have a desk job, but leave my desk regularly to run errands, greet visitors,
attend meetings, etc. at least _____ times an hour.

I engage in light sports activities (doubles tennis, softball, volleyball, social
dancing) _____ hours a week.

I engage in vigorous exercise _____ times a week for _____ minutes each time.

Please list your fitness goals: _____

Why are these goals important to you? _____

_____

How long do you think it will take to achieve these goals? _____

How committed are you to improving your fitness at this time? _____

What are your favorite exercise activities? _____

_____

What types of exercise have you tried in the past? _____

Have you had any negative exercise experiences? _____

Nutrition and Weight Profile

Name: _____ Date: _____

What is your current weight? _____ What would you like to weigh? _____

If you are trying to lose weight:

    What is the most you have weighed as an adult? _____

    What is the least you have weighed as an adult? _____

    How long did you maintain this weight? _____

    What is the lowest weight you have maintained for a year? _____

    How many times have you lost and regained weight? _____

    What types of diets have you tried? _____

    If you have high blood pressure or high cholesterol, at what weight did these problems develop? _____

    Do you have parents or siblings who are overweight?   Yes ❑ No ❑

    Is this a good time in your life to commit to a weight loss program (think about possible pressing responsibilities, unusual stressors or distractions, etc.)?   Yes ❑ No ❑

    What obstacles are in the way of achieving your goal? _____

Which do you eat regularly (check all that apply):

    ❑ Breakfast   ❑ Midafternoon snack

    ❑ Midmorning snack   ❑ Dinner

    ❑ Lunch   ❑ After-dinner snack

How often do you eat out each week? _____ times

What size portions do you normally have?

    ❑ Small   ❑ Moderate   ❑ Large   ❑ Extra-large   ❑ Uncertain

How often do you eat more than one serving?

    ❑ Always   ❑ Usually   ❑ Sometimes   ❑ Never

How long does it usually take you to eat a meal? _____ minutes

Do you eat while doing other activities (e.g., watching TV, reading, working)?
                                       Yes ❑ No ❑

How many times a week do you eat or drink the following?

    _____   cookies, cake, pie

    _____   candy

    _____   doughnuts

    _____   ice cream

_____ commercial muffins

_____ soft drinks

_____ potato chips, corn chips, etc.

_____ fried foods

_____ peanut butter, nuts or seeds

_____ crackers

_____ fast food (McDonald's, Taco Bell, etc.)

_____ cheese

_____ whole milk, cream, non-dairy creamer

_____ red meat (beef, pork, lamb)

_____ butter, margarine, mayonnaise

_____ breakfast meat or luncheon meat (bacon, sausage, hot dogs, salami)

_____ convenience items (frozen foods, instant products, canned soup, etc.)

_____ refined grains (e.g., white rice & breads) vs. whole grain

_____ more than one serving of alcohol daily (4 oz. wine, 1.5 oz liquor, 12 oz. beer)

_____ more than two servings of a caffeinated beverage in a day

How many servings of the following foods do you eat each day:

_____ fruit (1 small whole, or ½ cup)

_____ vegetables (½ cup)

_____ bread (1 slice)

_____ cereal (½ cup)

_____ pasta, rice, other grain (½ cup)

_____ dairy product (½ cup)

_____ meat (3 oz.)

_____ dried beans, peas, tofu, etc. (½ cup)

Self-Assessment Quiz

The following questionnaire is designed to increase your knowledge and awareness of your overall health, and to highlight potential areas of concern. It doesn't pinpoint how you compare to the rest of the population, but the scoring chart at the end will show you areas where you are making healthy choices and where there is room for improvement. Keep in mind that although health risks associated with age, gender, and heredity are beyond your control, you can modify a range of other factors, such as blood pressure, smoking, blood cholesterol levels, exercise, diet, stress, and excess body weight.

Section A: PHYSICAL FITNESS

1. Do you exercise or play a sport for at least thirty minutes three or more times a week? Yes ❑ No ❑

2. Do you warm up and cool down by stretching before and after exercising? Yes ❑ No ❑

3. Do you fall into the appropriate weight category for someone your height and gender? Yes ❑ No ❑

4. In general, are you pleased with the condition of your body? Yes ❑ No ❑

5. Are you satisfied with your current level of energy? Yes ❑ No ❑

6. Do you use stairs rather than escalators or elevators whenever possible? Yes ❑ No ❑

NUMBER OF ANSWERS EACH COLUMN ____ ____

Section B: FAMILY HISTORY

Do you have a grandparent, parent, aunt, uncle, brother, or sister who:

1. Had a heart attack before age forty? No ❑ Yes ❑

2. Had high blood pressure requiring treatment? No ❑ Yes ❑

3. Developed diabetes? No ❑ Yes ❑

4. Developed glaucoma? No ❑ Yes ❑

5. Developed gout? No ❑ Yes ❑

6. Developed breast cancer? No ❑ Yes ❑

NUMBER OF ANSWERS EACH COLUMN ____ ____

Section C: **SELF-CARE AND MEDICAL CARE**

1. Do you floss your teeth daily? Yes ❏ No ❏
2. Do you have a dental checkup at least one a year? Yes ❏ No ❏
3. Do you use sunscreen regularly and avoid extensive exposure to the sun? Yes ❏ No ❏
4. For women: do you examine your breasts for unusual changes or lumps at least once a month? Yes ❏ No ❏
5. For men: do you examine your testicles for unusual changes or lumps at least once every three months? Yes ❏ No ❏
6. Do you usually know what to do in case of illness or injury? Yes ❏ No ❏
7. Do you avoid unnecessary X-rays? Yes ❏ No ❏
8. Do you normally get an adequate amount of sleep? Yes ❏ No ❏
9. Have you had your blood pressure checked in the past year? Yes ❏ No ❏
10. For women: have you had a Pap smear within the last two years? Yes ❏ No ❏
11. If you are over forty: have you had a test for glaucoma within the last four years? Yes ❏ No ❏
12. If you are over forty: have you had a test for hidden blood in your stool within the last two years? If you are over fifty: within the last year? Yes ❏ No ❏
13. If you are over fifty: have you had a least one endoscopic exam of the lower bowel? Yes ❏ No ❏

NUMBER OF ANSWERS EACH COLUMN ____ ____

Section D: **EATING HABITS**

1. Do you drink enough fluids so that your urine is a pale yellow color? Yes ❏ No ❏
2. Do you try special or fad diets? No ❏ Yes ❏
3. Do you add salt to foods during cooking and at the table? No ❏ Yes ❏
4. Do you minimize your intake of sweets, especially candy and soft drinks, and avoid adding sugar to foods? Yes ❏ No ❏
5. Is your diet well-balanced (including vegetables, fruits, breads, cereals, dairy products, and adequate sources of protein)? Yes ❏ No ❏
6. Do you limit your intake of saturated fats (butter, cheese, cream, fatty meats)? Yes ❏ No ❏

7. Do you limit your intake of cholesterol
(eggs, liver, meats)?   Yes ❏ No ❏

8. Do you eat fish and poultry more often than red meats?   Yes ❏ No ❏

9. Do you eat high-fiber foods (vegetables,
fruits, whole grains) several times a day?   Yes ❏ No ❏

NUMBER OF ANSWERS EACH COLUMN   ____ ____

Section E: **ALCOHOL, NICOTINE, AND OTHER DRUG USE**

1. Do you smoke cigarettes, cigars, or a pipe,
chew tobacco, or use other drugs?   No ❏ Yes ❏

2. Do you limit yourself to no more than two drinks a day?   Yes ❏ No ❏

3. Have family members or friends ever commented
on or complained about your drinking or your
use of other drugs?   No ❏ Yes ❏

4. Have you been unable to recall things you did
when you are drinking or using other drugs?   No ❏ Yes ❏

5. Do you use alcohol or other drugs as a way of
handling stressful situations or problems in your life?   No ❏ Yes ❏

6. Do you read and follow the label directions when
using prescribed and over-the-counter drugs?   Yes ❏ No ❏

NUMBER OF ANSWERS EACH COLUMN   ____ ____

Section F: **ACCIDENTS**

1. Do you drive after drinking alcohol or using
other drugs, or ride with drivers who have been
drinking or using other drugs?   No ❏ Yes ❏

2. Do you obey traffic rules and stay within the
speed limit when you drive?   Yes ❏ No ❏

3. As a driver and passenger, do you wear a
seat belt at all times?   Yes ❏ No ❏

4. Are the vehicles you drive well-maintained?   Yes ❏ No ❏

5. Do you smoke in bed?   No ❏ Yes ❏

6. Are you informed and careful when using potentially harmful products or substances, such as household cleaners, poisons, flammables, solvents, and electrical devices?   Yes ❑ No ❑

7. Do you own a gun?   No ❑ Yes ❑

NUMBER OF ANSWERS EACH COLUMN ＿＿ ＿＿

Section G: **INTELLECTUAL LIFE, VALUES, AND SPIRITUALITY**

1. Are you interested in, and do you keep up to date on, social and political issues?   Yes ❑ No ❑

2. Are you satisfied with what you do for entertainment?   Yes ❑ No ❑

3. Do you engage in creative and stimulating activities as often as you would like?   Yes ❑ No ❑

4. Are you satisfied with the degree to which your work is consistent with your values?   Yes ❑ No ❑

5. Are you satisfied with the degree to which your leisure activities are consistent with your values?   Yes ❑ No ❑

6. Is it difficult for you to accept the values and life-styles of others when they are different from your own?   No ❑ Yes ❑

7. Are you satisfied with your spiritual life?   Yes ❑ No ❑

NUMBER OF ANSWERS EACH COLUMN ＿＿ ＿＿

Section H: **STRESS AND SOCIAL SUPPORT**

1. Are you satisfied with the amount of excitement in your life?   Yes ❑ No ❑

2. Do you find it easy to laugh?   Yes ❑ No ❑

3. Do you hold in your angry feelings without expressing them?   No ❑ Yes ❑

4. Do you make decisions with minimum stress and worry?   Yes ❑ No ❑

5. Do you include relaxation time as part of your daily routine?   Yes ❑ No ❑

6. Do you anticipate and prepare for events or situations likely to be stressful?   Yes ❑ No ❑

7. Have you had to make difficult readjustments at home or work in the past year?   Yes ❑ No ❑

8. Has a family member or close friend died, been seriously ill, or been injured within the past year?   No ☐   Yes ☐

9. Are you a chronic worrier, subject to guilt feelings or self-punishment?   No ☐   Yes ☐

10. Have your health, eating, or sleeping habits changed as a result of a stressful incident or situation during the past year?   No ☐   Yes ☐

11. Are you able to fall asleep when you are ready and to sleep through the night uninterrupted?   Yes ☐   No ☐

12. Do you wake up feeling rested?   Yes ☐   No ☐

13. Do you have one or more persons with whom you can discuss personal concerns, worries, or problems?   Yes ☐   No ☐

14. Do they make you feel respected and/or admired?   Yes ☐   No ☐

15. Is there someone to whom you can turn if you need help, such as to lend you money?   Yes ☐   No ☐

16. Are you satisfied with the support you provide to others?   Yes ☐   No ☐

NUMBER OF ANSWERS EACH COLUMN ____ ____

Section I: ENVIRONMENT

1. Are you often in an environment that has significant air and/or noise pollution?   No ☐   Yes ☐

2. Are you often exposed to asbestos, vinyl chloride, formaldehyde, or other toxins?   No ☐   Yes ☐

3. Do you miss many days at work due to illness or just not feeling up to it? ("Work" refers to daily activities, including school or work in the home.)   No ☐   Yes ☐

4. Do you often sit for periods of an hour or more at a time?   No ☐   Yes ☐

5. Are you satisfied with your ability to plan your workload?   Yes ☐   No ☐

6. Do you receive adequate feedback to judge your performance?   Yes ☐   No ☐

7. Are you satisfied with your balance between work and leisure time?   Yes ☐   No ☐

NUMBER OF ANSWERS EACH COLUMN ____ ____

Section J: **SEXUALITY**

1. Are you satisfied with your level of sexual activity? Yes ❏ No ❏
2. Are you satisfied with your sexual relationship? Yes ❏ No ❏
3. Are you satisfied with your use (or nonuse)
   of contraceptives? Yes ❏ No ❏
4. Are you satisfied with your use (or nonuse)
   of "safer sex" practices? Yes ❏ No ❏

NUMBER OF ANSWERS EACH COLUMN ____ ____

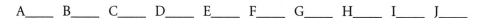

Scoring the Self-Assessment Quiz

For each section of the quiz, write the number of answers you marked in the left-hand column in the blanks below.

Sections:

A____   B____   C____   D____   E____   F____   G____   H____   I____   J____

In the circle graph below, shade in the number of subsections to correspond with the numbers you wrote above. Start with the innermost section. For example, if there are four answers marked in the left-hand answer column of Section D, that portion of the circle graph will look like this:

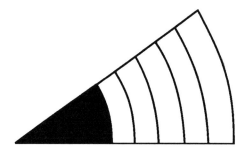

Sections that are completely shaded: you are making healthy behavior and life-style choices in these areas. Keep up the good work.

Sections that are partially shaded: with a little more awareness and effort in these areas, you could improve the quality of your life—and live longer.

Sections that are barely shaded or not shaded at all: there is significant room for increasing your health and satisfaction in these areas. Work first on those areas where you are most likely to be successful, then tackle the tougher sections.

Note: This grading system doesn't apply to section B since you have no control over your family history. If you answered "yes" to several questions about family history, try to compensate by concentrating on the other areas over which you do have control.

Excerpted from *The Wellness Encyclopedia,* © Health Letter Associates, 1991.

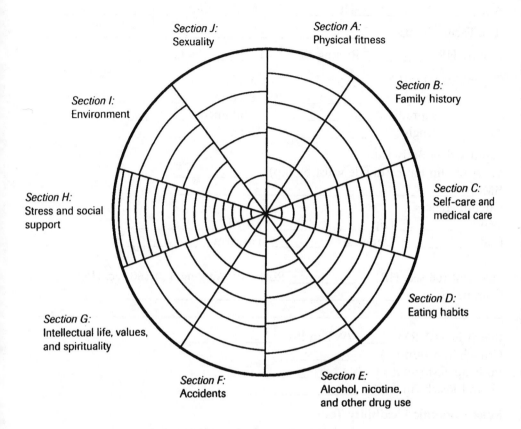

Section J:
Sexuality

Section A:
Physical fitness

Section B:
Family history

Section I:
Environment

Section C:
Self-care and
medical care

Section H:
Stress and social
support

Section D:
Eating habits

Section G:
Intellectual life, values,
and spirituality

Section F:
Accidents

Section E:
Alcohol, nicotine,
and other drug use

Excerpted from *The Wellness Encyclopedia*, © Health Letter Associates, 1991.

Fitness Assessment Data Sheet

Name _____ Date _____

Age_____ Wt_____ Ht _____   Medications _____

Risk Factor Status _____

Resting HR_____ Resting BP   (1) _____   (2) _____

Skinfolds: WOMEN   MEN
          Triceps   ___ ___ ___   Pectoral   ___ ___ ___
          Suprailiac ___ ___ ___   Abdomen ___ ___ ___
          Thigh   ___ ___ ___   Thigh   ___ ___ ___

Estimated % Body Fat
Waist to Hip Ratio (divide waist by hip) _____
BMI _____
Circumferences:
Waist_____ Hip _____ Thigh _____
Calf _____ Upper arms_____ Forearm_____

Step Test (60 sec. HR) _____ Rockport Walking Test (60 sec. HR)_____
Comments _____
_____

Bench Press 1 RM _____ /WT in lbs. _____ = _____
Crunch Test (#/min.) _____
Push-up Test (total #) _____
Sit and Reach (inches) _____

Muscle Specific Flexibility Tests

	Adequate	Needs improvement
Hamstrings	_____	_____
Iliopsoas	_____	_____
Quadriceps	_____	_____
Calves	_____	_____
Shoulders	_____	_____

Posture Assessments (visual)

	Yes	No
Lordosis	_____	_____
Kyphosis	_____	_____
Forward head	_____	_____
Hip height discrepancy	_____	_____
Shoulder height	_____	_____

Goal Setting Form

1. Rank your fitness/health goals

   #1 _____

   #2 _____

   #3 _____

2. How will goal #1 be achieved? (Consider frequency [list specific days & times], intensity, duration, mode, etc.) _____

   Goal #2?_____

   Goal #3?_____

3. Date for re-assessment _____

4. What, if any, dietary modifications need to be made (keep them achievable and realistic)?

   #1 _____

   #2 _____

   #3 _____

5. What obstacles might interfere with your goal achievement?

Obstacle	Strategy for overcoming obstacle
_____	_____
_____	_____
_____	_____

Behavior Contract

I, _____, am making a commitment to myself to
change the following behavior(s): _____
_____.

I agree to adhere to an exercise program for _____ weeks. I commit to exercising
_____ times per week and to increasing my overall level of physical activity. I
am doing this so that _____
_____.

I will reward myself by _____

Signed _____ Date _____

Witness _____ Date _____

Workout Log

Name: _____

Date	Cardio	Legs	Lats	Delts	Pecs	Traps & Rhomboids	Biceps	Triceps	Abs	Erector Spinae	Stretch	Other	Note

Endurance Activity—Progress Chart

Name: _____

Date															
Activity															
Program															
Duration															
Intensity															
Date															
Activity															
Program															
Duration															
Intensity															
Date															
Activity															
Program															
Duration															
Intensity															
Date															
Activity															
Program															
Duration															
Intensity															
Date															
Activity															
Program															
Duration															
Intensity															

Strength Conditioning

Name: _____

	Date				
LEG EXTENSION Seat Position #2	Pos. Wt.				
	Neg. Wt.				
	Reps.				
LEG CURL Seat Position #2	Pos. Wt.				
	Neg. Wt.				
	Reps.				
LEG PRESS Seat Position #2	Pos. Wt.				
	Neg. Wt.				
	Reps.				
CHEST PRESS Seat Position #2	Pos. Wt.				
	Neg. Wt.				
	Reps.				
FLY Seat Position #2	Pos. Wt.				
	Neg. Wt.				
	Reps.				
LAT PULL-DOWN Seat Position #2	Pos. Wt.				
	Neg. Wt.				
	Reps.				
SHOULDER PRESS Seat Position #2	Pos. Wt.				
	Neg. Wt.				
	Reps.				
SEATED ROW Seat Position #2	Pos. Wt.				
	Neg. Wt.				
	Reps.				
BACK EXTENSION Seat Position #4	Pos. Wt.				
	Neg. Wt.				
	Reps.				
ABDOMINAL Seat Position #4	Pos. Wt.				
	Neg. Wt.				
	Reps.				
ARM CURL Seat Position #4	Pos. Wt.				
	Neg. Wt.				
	Reps.				
TRICEPS EXTENSION Seat Position #4	Pos. Wt.				
	Neg. Wt.				
	Reps.				

Note: This program was designed to be used with the Lifecircuit system®.

Exercise Session Recording Form

Client Name _____ SS#_____ Date_____

Location _____ Time _____

Pre-exercise Client Affect

How do you feel? _____

How did you feel after last session? _____

_____

Exercise Session

I. Warm-up Component (Summary)

_____

_____

II. Cardiovascular Component

Target Heart Rate _____

Type of Ex.	Intensity	HR Response	Time	Client Response
_____	_____	_____	_____	_____
_____	_____	_____	_____	_____

III. Strength Component

Type of Ex.	Set	Reps	Weight	Client Response
1. _____	_____	_____	_____	_____
	_____	_____	_____	_____
	_____	_____	_____	_____
2. _____	_____	_____	_____	_____
	_____	_____	_____	_____
3. _____	_____	_____	_____	_____
	_____	_____	_____	_____
	_____	_____	_____	_____
4. _____	_____	_____	_____	_____
	_____	_____	_____	_____

5. _____ _____ _____ _____ _____

6. _____ _____ _____ _____ _____

7. _____ _____ _____ _____ _____

8. _____ _____ _____ _____ _____

IV. Cool-down Component (Summary of Cool-down Exercises and Client's Response)

General Summary of Session

Equipment Inventory Form

Equipment name	Type, (constant variable, etc.)	Number	Exercises that can be performed	Primary muscles worked
_____	_____	_____	_____	_____
_____	_____	_____	_____	_____
_____	_____	_____	_____	_____
_____	_____	_____	_____	_____
_____	_____	_____	_____	_____
_____	_____	_____	_____	_____
_____	_____	_____	_____	_____
_____	_____	_____	_____	_____
_____	_____	_____	_____	_____
_____	_____	_____	_____	_____
_____	_____	_____	_____	_____
_____	_____	_____	_____	_____
_____	_____	_____	_____	_____
_____	_____	_____	_____	_____
_____	_____	_____	_____	_____
_____	_____	_____	_____	_____
_____	_____	_____	_____	_____
_____	_____	_____	_____	_____
_____	_____	_____	_____	_____
_____	_____	_____	_____	_____

Appendix C
Fitness Norms

Percent Fat Estimations For Women

Age (years)

Sum of Three Skinfolds	18-22	23-27	28-32	33-37	38-42	43-47	48-52	53-57	>57
8–12	8.0	9.0	9.2	9.4	9.5	9.7	9.9	10.1	10.3
13–17	10.8	10.9	11.1	11.3	11.5	11.7	11.8	12.0	12.2
18–22	12.6	12.8	13.0	13.2	13.4	13.5	13.7	13.9	14.1
23–27	14.5	14.6	14.8	15.0	15.2	15.4	15.6	15.7	15.9
28–32	16.2	16.4	16.6	16.8	17.0	17.1	17.3	17.5	17.7
33–37	17.9	18.1	18.3	18.5	18.7	18.9	19.0	19.2	19.4
38–42	19.6	19.8	20.0	20.2	20.3	20.5	20.7	20.9	21.1
43–47	21.2	21.4	21.6	21.8	21.9	22.1	22.3	22.5	22.7
48–52	22.8	22.9	23.1	23.3	23.5	23.7	23.8	24.0	24.2
53–57	24.4	24.4	24.6	24.8	25.0	25.2	25.3	25.5	25.7
58–62	25.7	25.9	26.0	26.2	26.4	26.6	26.8	27.0	27.1
63–67	27.1	27.2	27.4	27.6	27.8	28.0	28.2	28.3	28.5
68–72	28.4	28.6	28.7	28.9	29.1	29.3	29.5	29.7	29.8
73–77	29.6	29.8	30.0	30.2	30.4	30.6	30.7	30.9	31.3
78–82	30.9	31.0	31.2	31.4	31.6	31.8	31.9	32.1	32.3
83–87	30.0	32.2	32.4	32.6	32.7	32.9	33.1	33.3	33.5
88–92	33.1	33.3	33.5	33.7	33.8	34.0	34.2	34.4	34.6
93–97	34.2	34.4	34.5	34.7	34.9	35.1	35.2	35.4	35.6
98–102	35.1	35.3	35.5	35.7	35.9	36.0	36.2	36.6	36.7
103–107	36.1	36.2	36.4	36.6	36.8	37.0	37.2	37.3	37.5
108–112	36.9	37.1	37.3	37.5	37.7	37.9	38.0	38.2	38.4
113–117	37.9	38.9	38.1	38.3	39.2	39.4	39.6	39.8	39.5
118–122	38.5	38.7	38.9	39.1	39.4	39.6	39.8	40.0	40.0
123–127	39.2	39.4	49.6	39.8	40.0	40.2	40.3	40.5	40.7
133–137	40.5	40.7	40.8	41.0	41.2	41.4	41.6	41.7	41.9
138–142	41.0	41.2	41.4	41.6	41.7	41.9	42.1	42.3	42.5
143–147	41.5	41.7	41.9	42.0	42.2	42.4	42.6	42.8	43.0
153–157	42.3	42.5	42.6	42.8	43.0	43.2	43.4	43.6	43.4
158–162	42.6	42.8	42.0	43.1	43.4	43.5	43.7	43.9	44.1
163–167	42.9	43.0	43.2	43.4	43.6	43.8	44.0	44.1	44.3
168–172	43.1	43.2	43.4	43.6	43.8	44.0	44.2	44.3	44.5
173–177	43.2	43.4	43.6	43.8	43.9	44.1	44.3	44.5	44.7
178–182	43.3	43.5	43.7	43.8	44.0	44.2	44.4	44.6	44.8

Jackson AS, Pollock ML: Tables determining relative body fat percent for men & women as reprinted from "Practical Assessment of Body Composition": Phys Sportsmed 1985: 13 (5): 76-90

Percent Fat Estimations For Men

Age (years)

Sum of Three Skinfolds	18–22	23–27	28–32	33–37	38–42	43–47	48–52	53–57	>57
8–12	1.8	2.6	3.4	4.2	4.9	5.7	6.5	7.3	8.1
13–17	3.6	4.4	5.2	6.0	6.8	7.6	8.4	9.1	9.9
18–22	5.4	6.2	7.0	7.8	8.6	9.3	10.1	10.9	11.7
23–27	7.1	7.9	8.7	9.5	10.3	11.1	11.9	12.6	13.4
28–32	8.8	9.6	10.4	11.2	12.0	12.8	13.5	14.3	15.1
33–37	10.4	11.2	12.0	12.8	13.6	14.4	15.2	15.9	16.7
38–42	12.0	12.8	13.6	14.4	15.2	15.9	16.7	17.5	18.3
43–47	13.5	14.3	15.1	15.9	16.7	17.5	18.3	19.0	19.8
48–52	15.0	15.8	16.6	17.4	18.1	18.9	19.8	20.5	21.3
53–57	17.8	18.5	19.3	20.1	20.9	21.7	22.5	23.3	24.1
58–62	19.1	19.9	20.6	21.4	22.2	23.0	23.8	24.5	25.4
63–67	20.3	21.1	21.9	22.7	23.5	23.8	25.1	25.8	26.6
68–72	21.5	22.3	23.1	23.9	24.7	25.5	26.3	27.0	27.8
73–77	22.7	23.5	24.3	25.0	25.8	26.6	27.4	28.2	29.0
78–82	23.8	24.6	26.4	27.2	28.0	28.8	29.6	30.3	31.1
83–87	24.8	25.6	26.4	27.2	28.0	28.8	29.6	30.3	31.1
88–92	25.8	26.6	27.4	28.2	29.0	29.8	30.5	31.3	32.3
93–97	26.7	27.5	28.3	29.1	29.9	30.7	31.5	32.3	33.4
98–102	27.6	28.0	29.2	30.0	30.8	31.6	32.4	33.2	33.9
103–107	28.5	29.3	30.1	30.8	31.6	32.4	33.2	34.0	34.8
108–112	29.3	30.0	30.8	31.6	32.4	33.2	32.0	34.8	35.6
113–117	30.0	30.8	31.6	32.4	33.1	33.9	34.7	35.5	36.3
118–122	30.7	31.5	32.3	33.0	33.8	34.6	35.4	36.2	37.0
123–127	31.3	32.1	32.9	33.7	34.4	35.2	36.0	36.8	37.6
133–137	31.9	32.7	33.4	42.2	45.0	35.8	36.6	37.4	38.2
138–142	32.4	33.6	34.4	35.2	36.0	36.8	37.6	38.4	39.2
143–147	32.9	33.6	34.4	25.2	36.0	36.8	37.6	38.4	39.2
148–152	33.3	34.1	34.8	35.6	36.4	37.2	38.0	38.8	39.6
153–157	33.6	34.4	35.2	36.0	36.8	37.6	38.4	39.2	39.9
158–162	33.9	34.7	35.5	36.3	37.1	37.9	38.7	39.5	40.3
163–167	34.2	35.0	35.8	36.3	37.4	38.1	38.9	39.7	40.5
168–172	34.4	35.2	36.0	36.8	37.6	38.4	39.1	39.9	40.7
173–177	34.6	35.3	36.1	36.9	37.8	38.5	39.2	40.1	40.9
178–182	34.7	35.4	36.2	37.0	37.8	38.6	39.4	40.2	42.1

Jackson AS, Pollock ML: Tables determining relative body fat percent for men & women as reprinted from "Practical Assessment of Body Composition": Phys Sportsmed 1985: 13 (5): 76-90

The Body Mass Index Nomogram

The Panel on Energy, Obesity, and Body Weight Standards has recommended that the following table be used when classifying obesity according to BMI values:

20–24.9 kg/m²	Desirable range for adult men and women
25–29.9 kg/m²	Grade 1 obesity
30–40 kg/m²	Grade 2 obesity
>40 kg/m²	Grade 3 obesity (morbid obesity)

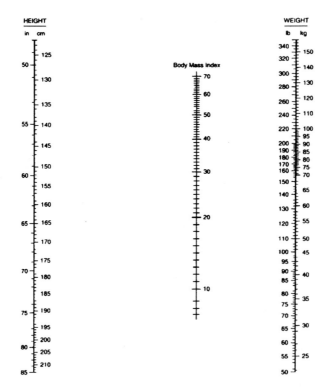

Note: The Body Mass Index (kg/m²) is calculated from the nomogram by reading the central scale after a straight edge is placed between height and body weight.

Reprinted with permission from Nieman, David C., *Fitness and Your Health*. Palo Alto, CA: Bull Publishing Co. 1993.

Norms for 3-Minute Step Test (Men)

Fitness Category	18–25	26–35	36–45	46–55	56–65	65+
			Age			
Excellent	<79	<81	<83	<87	<86	<88
Good	79–89	81–89	83–96	87–97	86–97	88–96
Above average	90–99	90–99	97–103	98–105	98–103	97–103
Average	100–105	100–107	104–112	106–116	104–112	104–113
Below average	106–116	108–117	113–119	117–122	113–120	114–120
Poor	117–128	118–128	120–130	123–132	121–129	121–130
Very poor	>128	>128	>130	>132	>129	>130

Adapted from the Y's Way to Physical Fitness (3rd ed.) by Golding, Larry, et al. With permission of the YMCA of the USA, 101 N. Walker Drive, Chicago, IL 60606.

Norms for 3-Minute Step Test (Women)

Fitness Category	18–25	26–35	36–45	46–55	56–65	65+
			Age			
Excellent	<85	<88	<90	<94	<95	<90
Good	85–98	88–99	90–102	94–104	95–104	90–102
Above average	99–108	100–111	103–110	105–115	105–112	103–115
Average	109–117	112–119	111–118	116–120	113–118	116–122
Below average	118–126	120–126	119–128	121–126	119–128	123–128
Poor	127–140	127–138	129–140	127–135	129–139	129–134
Very poor	>140	>138	>140	>135	>139	>134

Adapted from the Y's Way to Physical Fitness (3rd ed.) by Golding, Larry, et al. With permission of the YMCA of the USA, 101 N. Walker Drive, Chicago, IL 60606.

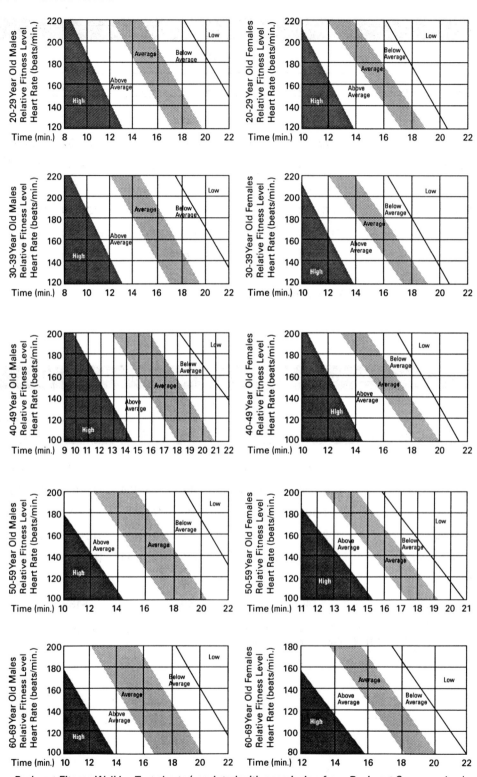

Rockport Fitness Walking Test charts (reprinted with permission from Rockport Company, Inc.)

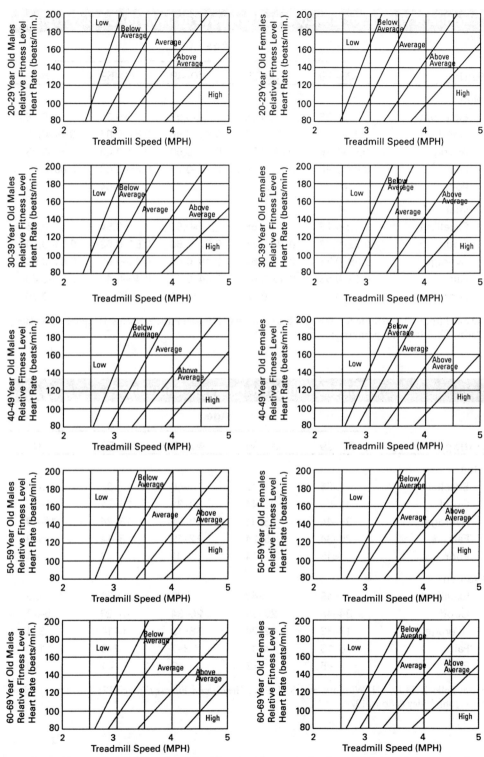

Rockport Fitness Tredmill Test charts (reprinted with permission from Rockport Company,Inc.)

Standard Values for Bench Press Strength in 1RM lb/lb Body Weight

	Age				
Rating	20–29	30–39	40–49	50–59	60+
Men					
Excellent	>1.26	>1.08	>0.97	>0.86	>0.78
Good	1.17–1.25	1.01–1.07	0.91–0.96	0.81–0.85	0.74–0.77
Average	0.97–1.16	0.86–1.00	0.78–0.90	0.70–0.80	0.64–0.73
Fair	0.88–0.96	0.79–0.85	0.72–0.77	0.65–0.69	0.60–0.63
Poor	<0.87	<0.78	<0.71	<0.64	<0.59
Women					
Excellent	>0.78	>0.66	>0.61	>0.54	>0.55
Good	0.72–0.77	0.62–0.65	0.57–0.60	0.51–0.53	0.51–0.54
Average	0.59–0.71	0.53–0.61	0.48–0.56	0.43–0.50	0.41–0.50
Fair	0.53–0.58	0.49–0.52	0.44–0.47	0.40–0.42	0.37–0.40
Poor	<0.52	<0.48	<0.43	<0.39	<0.36

Adapted from The Institute for Aerobics Research. 1985 Physical Fitness Norms. [Unpublished Data.] Dallas, TX, 1985, with permission.

Standard Values for Push-up Endurance

	Age				
Rating	20–29	30–39	40–49	50–59	60+
Men					
Excellent	>55	>45	>40	>35	>30
Good	45–54	35–44	30–39	25–34	20–29
Average	35–44	25–34	20–29	15–24	10–19
Fair	20–34	15–24	12–19	8–14	5–9
Poor	<19	<14	<11	<7	<4
Women					
Excellent	>49	>40	>35	>30	>20
Good	34–48	25–39	20–34	15–29	5–19
Average	17–33	12–24	8–19	6–14	3–4
Fair	6–16	4–11	3–7	2–5	1–2
Poor	<5	<3	<2	<1	<0

From Pollock, M.L., J.H. Wilmore, and S.M. Fox,: *Health and Fitness through Physical Activity.* New York: John Wiley & Sons, 1978.

Standard Values for Trunk Flexion in Inches

Rating	20–29	30–39	40–49	50–59	60+
Men					
Excellent	>22	>21	>20	>19	>18
Good	19–21	18–20	17–19	16–18	15–17
Average	13–18	12–17	11–16	10–15	9–14
Fair	10–12	9–11	8–10	7–9	6–8
Poor	<9	<8	<7	<6	<5
Women					
Excellent	>24	>23	>22	>21	>20
Good	22–23	21–22	20–21	19–20	18–19
Average	16–21	15–20	14–19	13–18	12–17
Fair	13–15	12–14	11–13	10–12	9–11
Poor	<12	<11	<10	<9	<8

Reprinted from Y's Way to Physical Fitness (3rd ed.) by Golding, Larry, et al. With permission of the YMCA of the USA, 101 N. Walker Drive, Chicago, IL 60606.

Norms for Abdominal Crunch Test (1 Min.)

Rating	20–29	30–39	40–49	50–59	60+
Men					
Excellent	>75	>75	>75	>74	>53
Good	41–74	46–74	67–74	45–73	26–52
Average	27–40	31–45	39–66	27–44	16–25
Fair	20–26	19–30	26–38	19–26	6–15
Poor	4–19	0–18	13–25	0–18	0–5
Women					
Excellent	>70	>55	>50	>48	>40
Good	37–69	34–54	34–49	23–47	23–39
Average	27–36	21–33	25–33	9–22	13–22
Fair	17–26	12–20	14–24	0–8	3–12
Poor	0–16	0–11	0–13	0	0–2

Based on data from Canadian Standardized Test of Fitness Operations Manual, 3rd. ed.(24)

Index

A

Accidents, 6
ACOG guidelines, 124
American College of Sports Medicine
    ACSM, 3, 15
    guidelines for resistance training, 78
    Position Stand, 48
    risk factors, 3
Actin, 75
Active listening, 116
Acute muscle soreness, 76-77
Aerobic capacity, 30
Aerobic or cardiorespiratory fitness, 30
AFAA 5 Questions, 89
Agreement and Release of Liability,
    17-18, 269
American Heart Association
    AHA, 93
    guidelines, 94
Amino acids, 94
Anaerobic power tests, 38
Anaerobic threshold, 30
Anorexia, 102-103
Antioxidants, 102
Arthritis, see osteoarthritis
Assessments
    body composition, 23, 26, 29, 45
    cardiorespiratory fitness, 23, 30
    flexibility, 23, 38-39, 45
    muscle endurance, 45
    muscle strength, 35, 45
    muscular strength/endurance, 23
Atherosclerosis, 2, 9, 125, 129

B

Back pain, 6, 38, 216
Back problems, 6
Back tests, 38
Ballistic stretching, 86
Behavior contract, 114, 294
Behavior modification, 110
Bench press strength, 308
Bench press test, 35-36
Benefits of
    cardiorespiratory fitness, 47
    fitness assessment, 22
    flexibility, 85
    muscular strength and endurance, 74
Blood pressure
    discussion of, 23-24
    measuring, 25
Body Mass Index (BMI), 26, 29, 104, 304
Bodybuilding, 223
Body composition assessment, 26-29
Bulimia, 103
Business aspects, 233

C

Caffeine, 22-24, 226
Calipers, 26-27
Caloric expenditure, 105-106
Cancer, 3-4, 8, 26, 93
Carbohydrates, 95, 100
Cardiorespiratory
    fitness, 30, 48, 50
    programming, 47
Case study, 19
Children, 229-230
Cholesterol, 3, 8, 42, 91, 95-97, 104
Cigarette smoking, 3

Initial interview, 14, 45
Injuries, 6, 219, 225
Intensity, 49-50, 87, 217
Interval training, 56-57
Isokinetic
    definition, 62
    resistance equipment, 80
    testing, 38
Isometric
    muscular contraction, 62
    resistance training, 81-82, 217
Isotonic, 62, 217

J

Joint
    actions, 61-62, 66-68
    movers, 62

K

Karvonen formula, 23, 50
Kinesiology, 59
Kyphosis, 42, 120-121

L

Label reading, 97
Legal considerations, 18-19
Liability insurance, 18
Lordosis, 42, 120-121
Low back pain, 5, 35, 37-38, 120

M

Marketing, 233
Maximal exercise tests, 30-31
Mechanism of injury, 223
Medical history forms, 15, 126, 278
METS, 51, 52-54
Minerals
    major, 99
    minor, 99
Mode, 55
Muscle
    atrophy, 228
    endurance, 35, 74, 77
    power, 77

soreness, 76
spindles, 75
terminology, 63
Myofibrils, 75
Myosin, 75

N

NIDDM, 128
Nutrient density, 99
Nutrition
    and weight management, 91
    and weight profile, 17, 282

O

Obesity, 3, 8-9, 91, 104
Olympic lifting, 223
One-repetition maximum (1 RM), 35
Order of exercises, 78
Osteoarthritis, 5
Osteoporosis, 5, 103
Overload, 48, 114, 218
Overtraining, 227-228

P

Periodization, 228
Physician's clearance, 16-17, 126
Physician's Clearance Form, 16-17, 280
Placebo effect, 225
Planes, 60-61
Plateau, 219
Plyometric training, 82
Postural screening, 40
Power lifting, 223
Pre- and post-exercise eating, 100
Pregnancy, 122-125
Pregnant, 15
Prevention, 1
Progression, 55-56, 79
Proper lifting techniques, 131-132
Proprioceptive neuromuscular facilitation,
    86-87
Proprioceptors, 75, 86
Protein, 93-94
Push-up test, 36, 308